EVERYTHING
YOU NEED TO KNOW
ABOUT MEDICAL
SCHOOL, RESIDENCY,
SPECIALIZATION,
AND PRACTICE

ON BECOMING A DOCTOR

TANIA HELLER, MD

FELLOW OF THE AMERICAN ACADEMY OF PEDIATRICS

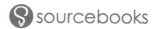

sourcebooks

Published by Sourcebooks, Inc.
P.O. Box 4410, Naperville, Illinois 60567-4410
(630) 961-3900
Fax: (630) 961-2168
www.sourcebooks.com

Library of Congress Cataloging-in-Publication Data

Heller, Tania
  On becoming a doctor : everything you need to know about medical school, residency, specialization, and practice / by Tania Heller.
      p. cm.
  Includes bibliographical references and index.
  1. Physicians--Vocational guidance. I. Title.
  R690.H4375 2009
  610.23--dc22
                      2009030716

Printed and bound in the United States of America.
POD 20 19 18 17 16 15 14 13 12 11

CONTENTS

PART THREE: REVIEW AND RESOURCES

ACKNOWLEDGMENTS

I am indebted to many people who have contributed to making this book a reality. Thank you to all the students and physicians who so kindly shared their stories with me. I would like to thank the Association of American Medical Colleges and the American Medical Student Association. I am also grateful to the experts I interviewed for their insight and valuable advice in regard to the medical school admissions process.

Thanks to Issy, Zelda, and Leon Heller for their input, and Sam, Daniel, and Ariel Messeca for their patience and support.

Note: Some names and identifying characteristics have been changed in order to maintain confidentiality.

PART ONE

PROLOGUE

FEBRUARY 5, 1978; 10 A.M.

Eight of us waited nervously outside the lab door in our starched white coats. We had heard horror stories of what awaited us. The stench of formaldehyde was unsettling. By the time we walked into the anatomy lab to dissect our first cadaver, only seven of us were still standing. Yet only four weeks later, prying apart the various organs, muscles, nerves, and vessels of the body assigned to us became so routine that all eight were able to discuss where we should have lunch after class.

CHAPTER 1

INTRODUCTION

As a student planning to enter medical school, you probably expect to take subjects that are at a far greater level of difficulty and intensity than those you took in college. However, some aspects of medical training, such as the dissection of human bodies, are a departure from anything that you faced as an undergraduate. Medical school will challenge you in many different ways—both intellectually and emotionally. "You're expected to know a lot and do a lot," said pediatrician Dr. Bertha Koomson. "You only appreciate the hard work and what you've learned later." My goal in writing this book is to provide you with information on the process of becoming a doctor, including medical school requirements and ways to finance your studies. You'll receive valuable tips and how-to advice from real doctors and medical students as well as other qualified individuals. You will have an inside look at the practice of medicine through interviews with specialists who describe their own exciting and varied experiences. Here, we will also examine the business side of a career in medicine. Numerous resources are included to help you navigate the process from start to finish.

WHAT INSPIRES YOUNG PEOPLE TO GO INTO MEDICINE?

My father taught me that our purpose in life is to leave the world a better place. Although I believe that to be true, I have asked myself, "What can one person do to make a difference?" As a physician, I think of famous people in the medical field—people like Drs. Salk and Sabin, who both discovered polio vaccines, and the cardiac surgeon Dr. Christiaan Barnard, who performed the first successful human heart transplant. Clearly, they made a difference, but can and should each one of us hope to achieve something as significant? Yes, as a physician you will be able to make a contribution and influence people's lives, even if your name doesn't go down in the history books.

There are doctors who have had a big impact on my life, people who have touched my heart, even though they may not know it. I'll always remember the emergency room doctor who treated my son's elbow injury with great skill and the internist who showed compassion when my grandmother was hospitalized. I'll never forget the neurologist who offered reassurance and support when I worried unnecessarily about a symptom I had. In every field and every walk of life, there are ways that each one of us can make a difference. The practice of medicine is one of those fields in which we have enormous opportunity to do just that.

When I was sixteen years old, I considered a future in either science or education. Many years later I was able to combine the two by pursuing a medical career and becoming a physician, enjoying practicing clinical medicine as well as lecturing on medical topics. I attended the University of Cape Town in South Africa and did clinical rounds at Groote Schuur Hospital, where the famous cardiac surgeons, the Barnard brothers, operated. I intended to practice medicine in that region.

However, life takes many interesting turns. Because of the political climate, our family immigrated to the United States, and I did my residency training in pediatrics at Georgetown University Medical Center in Washington, D.C. Somehow, things seemed to work out, and I've never looked back. I've always appreciated the fact that I had exposure to "third world" medicine and the medical needs in Africa, an experience that has served me well. For example, when one of my first young patients in the United States had tuberculosis, I was able to recognize his clinical symptoms and radiological findings more readily.

Next, several others will speak about their own reasons for choosing a medical career.

Wanting to Make a Discovery

"I was always interested in trying to discover things," said Dr. Roscoe Brady, who became a world-renowned scientist at the National Institutes of Health. "As a child, Edison was my hero, and my favorite book was *The Life of Thomas Edison*." Dr. Brady was the first of several people I interviewed about their choice to pursue a medical career. He told me that his father had been a pharmacist who made remedies and that some of his father's remedies are actually still in use to this day.

Wanting to Make a Difference in People's Lives

"I don't know if I could do it all over again," said Dr. Marc Simon, a cardiologist at a large academic medical center in Pittsburgh. "In other words, if I knew then, going forward, that I'd have to commit to so many years of training, I might not have made the decision to go into medicine. Now that I have completed my training, I am happy that I did."

Dr. Simon wanted to go into "the sciences" but didn't know whether he would proceed into the medical field. "I studied bioengineering in undergraduate school at the University of Pennsylvania," he told me. "My parents encouraged me to explore the medical field. During the summers, I worked in a lab with an oncologist (cancer specialist) who became my role model and was the greatest influence on my career choice. While that mentor ran a basic research laboratory in which I and so many other students worked, he was incredibly dedicated to his patients. I saw this firsthand on clinical rounds with him and in one-on-one discussions we would have both at work and at times when he would drive me home. We would discuss ethics, biology, and, occasionally, science. He was first and foremost a humanist. I discovered that I enjoyed going on clinical rounds, so I applied to medical school and was accepted to the University of Maryland."

Dr. Simon found that while science was a strong driving force, it was witnessing the tangible, positive effect on people's lives that he most enjoyed. "For me, medicine is both about the patients and the science of improving their—and future patients'—lives," he said. "It is a special privilege and honor to be involved in both clinical medicine and research that took me many extra years of training." He told me that despite difficult years, he made the right career choice in academic medicine. "I can't imagine doing anything else."

Interest in Science as Well as Personal Interaction

Ari Kestler, a second-year medical student, recounted his experience to me. Like his father, he was fascinated by science, and in high school he considered pursuing a medical degree. "I played hockey and my coach was a senior at [the University of] Maryland planning to go to medical school. He became my mentor in high school and college."

As a biochemistry major at the University of Michigan, Ari found his professors to be passionate and supportive of his interest, encouraging him to study hard and do research. At that time he considered pursuing a PhD, but after two summers in the confinement of a laboratory, he soon realized he needed more personal contact and took the Medical College Admission Test (MCAT) in the hopes of becoming a doctor.

Fascination with the Human Body

Avital Perry serves in the Israeli Defense Forces. She completed her undergraduate degree at the University of Maryland and has been accepted to an Ivy League medical school. "I considered law," she said. "I was argumentative and loved debating issues. Then, in high school, I studied biology, and the more I learned, the more I wanted to know. Science and particularly the study of the human body were fascinating to me. I liked laboratory work and enjoyed critical thinking. To see if I was capable of working with sick patients, I volunteered to assist in hospitals, including an intensive care neurosurgery unit where the Israeli Prime Minister later became a patient. I got to observe great doctors and nurses and had exposure to really ill people."

Avital told me that during her senior year, she volunteered at the FDA (Food and Drug Administration) in Bethesda, Maryland. "It was important for me to see what research was like, and I spent about forty hours a week there for most of that period. Though it was interesting, it was not what I wanted to do for a career. My bachelor's degree was in neuroscience, and in Israel I had a chance to work with some of the best neurosurgeons. I am currently leaning towards neurosurgery. There is so much that is unknown in terms of the human brain, and I believe there is opportunity for open-minded young doctors to enter this cutting-edge field." Now, Avital is sure that medicine is the right career for her. "I am very competitive," she said. "I love asking questions and trying to figure things out."

Father Was a Role Model

"I can't picture myself doing anything else. This is who I am," said Dr. Sandra Roberts. Ever since middle school, she knew that she wanted to be a physician. Her father was a general practitioner who had a small office attached to their home. As a teenager she thumbed through his books on anatomy, physiology, and dermatology, mesmerized by the drawings and photographs. She grew up listening to the advice that he gave his loyal patients and their families. He treated his patients with kindness and respect, and in turn, they respected him.

Fascinated with medicine, she was clear about her future path. She went on to graduate and then specialize in obstetrics and gynecology as an attending physician in a large teaching hospital. She is well aware that the practice of medicine today is very different from what it was years ago when her father practiced alongside their home. Now it is less personal and involves more administrative responsibility, but she is still happy with her decision to go into this field.

IS THERE A DOCTOR IN YOUR HOUSE?

I was interested but not surprised to discover a recurring theme in my interviews with medical students and physicians. Although this is not always the case, time after time I heard that inspiration came from a parent—in these interviews, several had parents who were doctors. A significant percentage had fathers, and a smaller percentage, mothers, who were physicians. I believe this will change in the near future as the number of women going into medicine has increased. Several of those interviewed told me that they grew up being exposed to the medical field, and it seemed inevitable they would follow that path. Others grew up in a medical environment, but it took a mentor to inspire them to pursue a medical career. But do not be disheartened if you don't have a doctor in the family. Many physicians, including me, did not have a parent in the field and pursued medicine anyway.

Our field is exciting and rapidly evolving. Significant discoveries with respect to the human genetic makeup have led to advances in the understanding and treatment of countless diseases. Advancement in technology has led to more rapid diagnosis and treatment options such as microscopic surgery, and the ability to obtain and share medical knowledge is easier and quicker in this electronic age. In the near future, the nature of professional practice will be dramatically different.

In spite of these breakthroughs and the explosion of readily available information, there are still concerns. There is no doubt that diagnostic studies (if used judiciously) can save lives. However, I worry that we physicians may lose some of our clinical skills if we rely too heavily on technology, neglecting critical thinking abilities (i.e., analyzing and interpreting) and clinical judgment. Other problems include the rising costs of health care and the lack of universal access to care in many countries. The malpractice crisis, caused by a significant number of lawsuits—both legitimate and frivolous—sometimes leads to unnecessary diagnostic testing in order to avoid missing a disease and being sued. Recent advances have also led to increased specialization, which is necessary to a certain extent, but the danger of which is poor continuity of care. We already have an insufficient number of primary care physicians.

We could do better in terms of preventing problems such as substance abuse, teenage pregnancy, and obesity, each with their own complications. On the positive side, however, our capability for treatment and prevention of disease (largely due to immunization) has expanded, and as a future doctor, your medical career choices are greater than ever before. You will see that practicing medicine can be as diverse as treating children or the aged, performing complicated heart procedures, delivering babies, discovering a cure for cancer, or even working in counterterrorism.

In this chapter, you have heard doctors and students describe their own reasons for entering the field of medicine. In the next chapter, we will explore whether medicine is the right career for you.

CHAPTER 2

IS MEDICINE THE CAREER FOR YOU?

There are some people who know exactly what they want to do even before entering high school. The aspiring actor who has visualized himself on Broadway, the would-be chef who has grown up watching the cooking channel, and the future biologist who collected fireflies as a child and remains fascinated by all living creatures—these are the fortunate few.

Most are uncertain of their career paths, even after completing high school or college. They may begin in one field and then change course along the way. In fact, later in this book, you will read about a doctor who started off as a musician and then graduated from medical school and pursued a successful career in pathology. Sometimes doctors give up their medical careers temporarily or permanently to raise children or become writers or lawyers. Next, read about the path Ryan took before he discovered what he really wanted to do.

RYAN'S STORY

Premedical student Ryan Curfiss graduated with a degree in engineering and then, after working for a few years, gave up that career to pursue medicine. "Medicine is something I've always thought about," said Ryan. "I enjoyed reading anatomy books and studying biology even in high school. The field always fascinated me, but when I imagined all that extra work, the many years of study, and the cost of training, I put the idea aside. Instead, I applied and was accepted to Virginia Tech as an undergraduate student in civil engineering. After graduating, I worked as project manager for construction companies for several years, but although I enjoyed the people, I didn't get the job satisfaction I was hoping for." Ryan said that the longer he waited, the more convinced he became that engineering was not for him. Now, he wishes he had applied to medical school sooner.

"My parents' neighbor was an engineer who later became an emergency room physician," said Ryan. "He was the one who made me realize that this was possible. I met with an advisor at Virginia Commonwealth University (VCU), and he guided me through the process, including which courses I needed to take. Last fall I entered the postbaccalaureate premedical program at VCU, and I hope to have all my undergraduate requirements completed by the summer." Ryan plans to take the MCAT exam in summer and apply to medical school in the fall.

I asked whether there had been anyone or anything else that had inspired him to consider medicine. "My earliest significant exposure to medicine was as a patient," he said. "I was admitted to the hospital with septic bursitis. The treatment course was complicated, and I required surgery and several weeks of rehabilitation. It was an intense introduction to the world of medicine." On the other hand, Ryan told me he found the experience interesting, even as he lay in bed "watching his knee swell". He continued, "I enjoyed talking to my orthopedist, and I am currently considering orthopedics as an option."

Ryan also works with the volunteer rescue squad and is currently in the process of becoming an emergency medical technician (EMT). "My first night on call began very quietly," he said. "I had been at the station for eight hours. Suddenly, at 2:00 a.m., we received an emergency call. A man had driven his car into a telephone pole and was knocked unconscious. We rushed to the scene and had to cut the vehicle into two pieces so that we could remove him through the backseat." Ryan then explained that not all situations are as dramatic. "Most of the calls are for patients who are not in life-threatening situations, but need to get to the hospital quickly. The most important thing for me is, at the end of the day, I really feel as if I'm helping people." For that reason, Ryan advises students to volunteer on a rescue squad. "You certainly get to see it all," he said.

Ryan is now a twenty-seven-year-old former engineer who has sold his home and given up his career to pursue a dream. He told me that it was nerve-racking to start over, but then he said something that put it all into perspective and made me believe he was on the right path. "Last night I worked with the rescue squad all night," he said. "I got home at eight o'clock this morning, and although I was exhausted, I felt as if I could keep going. When I finish my duty with the squad, I count the days until I can go back."

BUT WHAT IF YOU'RE STILL NOT SURE?

Ryan realized his passion, but how do you decide on a career path and whether medicine is an option for you? You will first need to take stock of your own values, what you enjoy doing, and what you do well.

If you are thinking about a future in medicine, it is important that you understand what you're getting yourself into. The medical field is very broad. You have options even if you don't want to have direct patient contact. However, if you intend to be involved in patient care, you should definitely be comfortable around sick people.

Spend time working in the healthcare field—perhaps alongside a doctor in an office, clinic, or hospital setting—while you are in high school or college. There is so much you can learn from watching and listening to professionals in those environments. One student told me that because he had a front desk job in a medical center, he learned a lot about patient care. In our private pediatric practice, we had medical students rotate through our office on a regular basis. The more enthusiastic, knowledgeable, and committed the students were, the more responsibility we gave them. After spending a month or two with us, many students had a good idea about whether they wanted to consider a career in pediatrics or not. Students who succeed are not only hardworking and persevering, but have a deep desire to learn as well as help and heal others. If you possess these qualities and have good communication skills, medicine may well be the right career choice for you.

One doctor I interviewed told me that it was always her ambition to practice medicine. She was told by her family that it could not happen, she would never achieve her goal, it was beyond her reach. No one in her family had even made it to graduate school. She heard she was neither smart enough nor wealthy enough. Although disheartened, she trusted her instincts, pursued a medical career, and achieved great success. It seems that if you believe in yourself, like the subject matter, know how to study, and have the passion to be a doctor, you can succeed. Set priorities so that you can achieve your goals and follow your dream.

DO YOU HAVE THE QUALITIES OF A GOOD DOCTOR?

It should go without saying that physicians should have integrity and be compassionate. In this section, we will discuss other attributes that may contribute to the making of a good doctor. I asked several physicians for their opinions.

Being Current

"It's important to stay on top of what's going on in medicine scientifically," said Dr. Maria Mannarino. "Doctors must continually update themselves about medications, new treatments, and other advances in medicine—that means reading books and articles and attending meetings—throughout your career. They also need to really talk to the patient to elicit a proper history in order to make an accurate diagnosis and good treatment plan. Some doctors spend too much of their time at the computer and too little with the patient."

Listening Well

Fortunately, many characteristics of good doctors can be learned or developed with experience, but there are still personality traits that suit certain specialties. "You certainly can do a better job if you tend to be a good listener, are willing to spend time with people, and don't need instant gratification," said Dr. Carol Salzman about internists.

Being Comfortable Dealing with Various Situations

Dr. Craig Futterman, a pediatric intensive care specialist, described the contrast between primary care medicine and intensive care. These specialties involve very different lifestyles and practice environments, and candidates should feel comfortable dealing with the types of situations each present. "Whereas in general pediatrics most of what one does is routine, and every now and then you see something unexpected," said Dr. Futterman, "in my field you get the unexpected most of the time, and only once in a while you see something routine. There is nothing mundane about what goes on in my life."

Ability to Remain Calm

For those students considering the pursuit of anesthesiology, Dr. Michael Jach said, "If you are a nervous or anxious person, don't go into anesthesiology. In this field, there's no room for panic." And the same holds true for specialties such as surgery, emergency room medicine, and psychiatry.

Being Detail-Oriented

With respect to pediatrics, although it goes without saying that it is important to like children, Dr. Lisa Crim added, "Pediatricians should be detail-oriented, because little things can easily be missed, and in children, they really count."

Knowledge and Curiosity

Being knowledgeable is an essential attribute of a good doctor, but it isn't enough. One has to be intellectually curious, analytical, and determined to look deeper when a diagnosis doesn't present itself clearly or immediately.

Persistence

Frequently, one has to be persistent in order to come up with answers.

Skilled at Communication

In many specialties, doctors must also have good communication skills. They need to convey information clearly to the patient so that it is understood. Giving a diagnosis is not enough. If the patient has a poor understanding of the illness, its treatment, and its implications, the treatment may be sidetracked.

Luckily, the doctor-patient relationship is being emphasized more in medical schools. I spoke to a therapist who teaches these skills to students, and she said that good doctors "listen and also remember their patients' stories."

Empathy

Another important quality for a physician is empathy. Being able to put yourself in the shoes of a patient and care about that person's well-being is key to a good doctor-patient relationship.

Critical Thinking

Medicine is both science and art. One has to incorporate a significant amount of information and put it into context. Diagnostic studies are extremely useful, but two physicians can be presented with the same diagnostic information about a patient, and they may each interpret and apply it differently. For example, a patient with weight loss and anemia could have an infectious disease, depression resulting in poor nutrition, an eating disorder, or cancer, among other things. It takes an astute physician to consider a broad differential diagnosis and explore the appropriate avenues.

SACRIFICE FOR A WORTHY CAUSE

Becoming a physician is challenging and requires significant sacrifice. The process will involve many years of training, including college, medical school, residency, and possibly a fellowship. You may incur substantial financial debt. Applying to medical school requires careful planning and preparation. You will need to take specific courses and become involved in extracurricular activities that could enhance your skills and help make you a well-rounded individual as early as middle or high school. Pursue activities that you enjoy and about which you feel passionate. Have some fun, too.

Later, consider the repercussions on your family life, and choose a partner who understands the stresses and demands of a medical career. If you are a parent in medical school, you will have to find a balance between spending time with your children and spending time in class and studying. With a greater number of households having two working parents, this has become more of an issue in recent years. The demands on a medical student's time can be overwhelming at times. You'll need understanding friends and a supportive home environment.

The rewards, on the other hand, are many. The study of medicine is vast, interesting, and forever-changing. Although doctors' salaries vary significantly among specialties, a medical career usually provides financial stability and security. There are so many opportunities available to physicians, with choices that include hospital work, private practice, public health, and scientific research. Most importantly, medicine is an honorable and respected profession in which one can derive great satisfaction by helping others.

We have now explored whether medicine may be the career for you, examined a few of the qualities that make a good doctor, and reminded ourselves of the sacrifices as well as the rewards of such a career. But once you have made the decision to pursue medicine, what is the next step you should take? In the following chapter, you will read more about the specific requirements for medical school.

CHAPTER 3

MEDICAL SCHOOL REQUIREMENTS

The next section reviews undergraduate course requirements as well as experience you should acquire both within and outside of the medical field, while also highlighting the value of mentorship.

REQUIRED UNDERGRADUATE COURSES

You will need to complete a minimum number of course credits and/or obtain a bachelor's degree prior to entering medical school. The requirements vary from school to school. Which school you attend for your undergraduate education really depends on what feels right to you and what makes you happy. For example, among other considerations, you need to decide whether you want to attend a larger state school or smaller, private one. You can obtain more information about the teaching staff and research opportunities at various schools by attending open houses, speaking to students and professors, or sitting in on classes.

Pre-medical students are not required to major in the sciences. However, although no specific major is required, as an undergraduate you will generally have to complete both science and nonscience courses before applying to medical school.

You should check each medical school's specific requirements with respect to number of course credits as well as laboratory experience. Admission requirements for some schools may include completion of specific courses such as biology, physics, chemistry and English. They may also require additional courses, e.g. biochemistry, statistics, calculus and behavioral sciences. Other schools use a competency-based admissions process instead. Your grade point average (GPA) will be an important factor in determining your acceptance to medical school, so getting good grades in college is essential. You will be able to find information on U.S. and Canadian medical school requirements in *Medical School Admission Requirements* (MSAR), which is produced by the AAMC and can be accessed online (see Resources in Part Three). Note that although medical school training generally spans four years, some medical schools in the U.S. provide programs of varying lengths that combine undergraduate (Baccalaureate) and M.D. training.

EXPERIENCE WITHIN THE MEDICAL FIELD

There are many opportunities for applicants to gain experience within the healthcare system. Susan and Katie provide two examples.

Susan, a high school junior with an ambition to become a doctor, volunteered in a clinic for underprivileged families the summer before her junior year. She was able to observe diagnostic and speech therapy sessions for the clinic's patients with developmental disabilities, including autism. In return, Susan helped with filing and paperwork for the clinic. She told me that in order to work in the clinic she had to sign a confidentiality statement and become certified in HIPAA (Health Insurance Portability and Accountability Act). "Working in the clinic was such a good experience," she said. "I had never before observed therapy sessions or those types of doctor-patient and parent-child interactions. I spent five weeks there and learned a lot." Susan then told me that she still goes to the clinic once a month. "They have a monthly support group for the mothers, and I help by setting up the room and taking care of the children."

Katie worked as an administrative assistant at a medical center during her second year in college. She scheduled appointments, filed charts, and accepted payments. When there was time, she took the opportunity to speak to the doctors and other staff and absorb as much medical information as she could.

As an applicant, it is important to demonstrate that you have gained experience and understanding of the profession by working or volunteering in the medical field, for example in clinics, physicians' offices, emergency centers, or hospitals. In order to make an informed decision about whether you want to enter this profession or not, it is also important that you know about the clinical and ethical issues physicians regularly face and have some understanding of the current healthcare system. Talk to your own physician or contact a local hospital to ask about volunteer or work opportunities.

Rather than simply "shadowing" a physician, get involved to whatever extent that you are able. Ask for responsibilities within reason. When you do apply to medical school you will describe your work and experience, and include the number of hours you spent in each situation. Explain what you learned from this opportunity and how it changed you as a person. Simply stating that you spent a certain number of days in a doctor's office is not going to set you apart from the many other applicants. The pathway to a medical degree is exciting and wonderful, but time-consuming as well. It is important that you are aware of the commitment you will make by choosing this path.

EXTRACURRICULAR EXPERIENCE

In addition to activities related to medicine, it is important to demonstrate that you are well-rounded by virtue of your extracurricular activities. You may, for example, join a club at school, either science-related or not (e.g., music, politics, art or sports). If these opportunities do not exist in your school, ask for permission to start your own club. You can also volunteer at your school or local community center. I know a student who spent most of her free time assisting young people with disabilities and also helped to raise money for sick children. If you have held a part-time job for a significant length of time, this can demonstrate responsibility and acquisition of knowledge in a specific field. Admission committees are looking for commitment and dependability. As an applicant, you will not only be evaluated on your academic achievements, but also on the basis of your ability to successfully lead a balanced life.

MENTORSHIP

Mentors are advisors and teachers who help with the guidance and development of a student, acting as an advocate when necessary. Most doctors can name people who taught, encouraged, and supported them at vital periods along the way to the establishment of their careers. Before, I may have taken my mentors for granted, but I now identify the ones who helped to shape my life as a doctor.

In medical school, my first mentor was a fellow student who had an affinity for chemistry. He joined our study group and raised the standard. When we thought we couldn't do any better, he knew we could, and so we did. He helped me by setting an example while also offering encouragement and friendship. During my clinical years, I was mentored by a colleague's father, who was a physician in private practice. A few classmates and I met with him regularly, reviewing subjects like pathology and discussing the application of the sciences to clinical medicine.

Later, during my residency, I was lucky enough to encounter another mentor, a pediatrician, who inspired me to work with and help children and teenagers. He had so much dedication and demonstrated such willingness to give of his valuable time to teach others, including me. During my early years in private practice, I was influenced by an emergency room physician, who was also a wonderful teacher. He gave me advice and left me with many clinical "pearls of wisdom" that I still find useful. He opened doors so that I could more easily reach my goals. One of my colleagues, a psychiatrist and author, inspired me to pursue writing. To this day, I still count all of them as my mentors. But that's my experience. Now read a student's point of view.

I had the opportunity to speak to Gabi, a junior in an elite high school for students with special aptitudes for the sciences. She spoke about the importance of mentors in her life. "Once a month I meet with a professor who works in academic medicine as well as private practice," she said. She told me that she plans to pursue a similar career, combining clinical medicine with research. "He is not only my teacher, but he is so inspiring to me. He has taught me about medicine and science, about responsibility, and has also guided me in regard to my own career path."

Gabi spoke about another one of her mentors, too. Students at her school are given a day each week to engage in research and work with scientists and physicians in various fields of study. They have an opportunity to find mentors within their areas of interest. "I was lucky," she said, "because I applied to work on an existing research study and was accepted. This is an ongoing, eight-year project on brain damage and its effect on language, and I will participate throughout this and next year. I work with my mentor, who is a PhD candidate. She gives me material to study and explains how the research is conducted." Gabi told me that before she transferred to this academy, she didn't know this whole world of science existed. She is planning to apply to an MD/PhD program and ultimately pursue a medical career.

Gabi advises every high school student to find a mentor. "I have found mine to be very helpful when I have needed contacts and resources. I am also going to ask for letters of recommendation for summer programs," she said. "Go to any university website and look at the projects they are working on. If you are interested, find the appropriate contacts and their email addresses. Another option is to write letters to doctors or scientists describing your interest in their field or research area. Whatever method you use—even if you contact a friend of a friend—try to make some connection to find a mentor or secure your program of preference."

The National Research Mentoring Network (NRMN) is a nationwide, NIH-funded program that connects undergraduates, graduates and postdocs pursuing biomedical research with mentors. The program promotes diversity in the research workforce and provides access for individuals from underrepresented and disadvantaged backgrounds to evidence-based mentoring.

For more information you may visit www.nrmnet.net.

It is important that you begin to build a network and associate with people who can encourage, support, and even protect you. Develop relationships with people within your field. Find good mentors who can guide and advise you. These may be students, counselors, lecturers, professors, or others who inspire you. Soon after writing this section of the book, I was asked to become a mentor for a student who was considering a medical career. I remembered how I valued the mentors in my life. It was an honor to offer my service to someone else.

GET SUPPORT

To be successful, you will need to have a strong support system. Even the most accomplished people don't achieve success by themselves. Support can come from family, friends, and peers who have your best interests at heart. Spend time with people who can encourage you but are not afraid to offer constructive criticism either. Without my parents' support, I may not have been able to pursue a medical career at all.

If you don't find the type of support you need from family or friends, there are other sources you can go to for help. Speak to a school counselor or a teacher you respect. They, too, may offer support and guidance.

INVESTING IN SUCCESS

Successful people are usually skilled at time management and able to set priorities. They also know that life has ups and downs, and the road to success is not always smooth. Those people who are able to manage stress and persevere even in challenging times have an advantage. Begin to develop the habits that can lead you to success. Get as much experience as you can, build a network of support, stay organized, allow time for relaxation and hobbies, but always remain focused on your goal.

If these skills don't come naturally, they can be learned. For example, keep an organizer with a list of both your short- and long-term goals. Then make a to-do list and prioritize. Each evening, take a few minutes to think about the most important tasks you need to accomplish the following day; then focus on those first. Learn to say no to insignificant requests, especially those that don't give you satisfaction.

We have reviewed medical school requirements and some of the skills that can enhance your success. In the next chapter, we will discuss the medical school application and the MCAT exam.

POSTBACCALAUREATE PROGRAMS

Some students choose to pursue a postbaccalaureate program (to improve their academic record or complete required pre-med courses) before applying to medical school.

A significant number of students take one or more 'gap years' between college and medical school to pursue activities such as work, study or research.

CHAPTER 4

Applying to Medical School and the MCAT Exam

This chapter delves into more of the specifics of the medical school application process and the MCAT.

MEDICAL COLLEGE ADMISSION TEST

A prerequisite for entry into virtually all U.S. medical schools is the Medical College Admission Test (MCAT), administered by the Association of American Medical Colleges (AAMC). The MCAT is a standardized, computer-based exam that tests knowledge of natural, behavioral and social sciences, as well as critical analysis and problem-solving skills. In addition to a total score, scores are reported for each of the four sections of the test. The MCAT exam undergoes periodic reviews to ensure that the content is such that the scores will be useful to admissions committees that are charged with selecting the best applicants. The most recent update in 2015 reflects the significant changes and advances in Medicine and health care.

The MCAT is administered multiple times a year. You should take it when you are ready and no later than the year in which you apply for medical school. Speak to a pre-health advisor to help you decide the best time for you.

You will need to register for the test online through the AAMC and then have your test scores sent with your medical school application. The scores of the MCAT are used as one of the major factors in deciding whether or not an applicant is admitted to a particular school. Although students can take the MCAT more than one time, it is best to approach the exam as if you will take it only once.

When preparing to take the MCAT, it is important to carefully read the information on the MCAT website. You should review your course material thoroughly for the test. There are numerous review books and excellent courses available to help you prepare for the MCAT. Taking the practice tests provided by these courses can be very beneficial and familiarize you with the format of the test. Another strategy that can be helpful is forming study groups rather than studying alone. You can obtain more information about the MCAT and the procedure involved in reporting scores to medical schools from college pre-medical advisors, online (at www.aamc.org), or by writing to the MCAT program directly.

I spoke to a college student and a medical student to get their takes on preparing for the MCAT exam. Later, they also commented on many other aspects of the application process.

Sam, our college student, is preparing to take the MCAT exam soon. He said that he will definitely sign up for an MCAT review course and believes that students who do so perform much better. Ari, our second-year medical student, also recommends a review course; however, he feels it really depends on the student. "If you have enough discipline to do the work on your own, you can study a review book instead."

MEDICAL SCHOOL APPLICATION

Undergraduate students should become familiar with the medical school admission process early in their college careers. Most U.S. MD-granting medical schools use the American Medical College Application Service (AMCAS), an AAMC service, for submitting the primary application. Participating public medical schools in Texas use the Texas Medical and Dental Schools Application Service (TMDSAS). AACOMAS is the online application service for U.S. Colleges of Osteopathic Medicine. Because the application can be time-consuming and confusing, visit the appropriate website in advance to review what is required. Although new application forms are released each year, they are generally quite similar. You can create a username and password that can be used for registering for the MCAT test as well as your medical school application through the American Medical College Application Service (AMCAS).

The AAMC produces *Medical School Admission Requirements* (MSAR) as well as the AMCAS instruction manual, which is available as a PDF document. Free of charge, this document explains the application process in detail. It will generally be faster to obtain information this way rather than by placing phone calls to the AAMC, as it receives a high volume of calls during the application period.

The application process can be very costly, especially if you apply to numerous schools, as many students do. The AAMC does run a Fee Assistance Program that can help eligible students offset some of the costs. If a fee assistance application is approved, the MCAT fee is reduced, the initial AMCAS fees (for one application) are forgiven, and a certain maximum number of medical school application fees are waived. These benefits may change. For more information, log on to the AAMC website at www.aamc.org.

A PANEL WEIGHS IN

I created a panel comprised of a college student, a medical student, a practicing physician, and a director of admissions at a medical school to weigh in on various aspects of the medical application process. Each spoke about his or her own experiences and gave insight from different vantage points. I asked them to comment on undergraduate courses and extracurricular requirements, as well as make any other recommendations for future students.

Sam, the third-year college student, started off as a nonscience major and then switched to neuroscience in his third year. He said that although he wasn't required to major in the sciences, it was a good decision for him. "It was important for me to learn more about health-related topics at that stage. It really tested my passion for medicine." According to a director of admissions at a well-known medical school, it is not necessary for students to major in the sciences. Instead, they should do what interests them, as long as they fulfill all the admission requirements and have an aptitude for the sciences.

With respect to extracurricular experience and work during the college years, Sam said that he was going to find a summer hospital volunteer position; however, he believed that the most important determining factors in acceptance to medical school were GPA and MCAT scores rather than extracurricular experience.

Current medical student Ari Kestler couldn't agree more. He believes that the best indicators as to whether one will succeed in the first few years of medical school are one's test scores and grades. In college, he "shadowed" physicians in private practice and in community settings, but he felt that most of the information went "over his head" so early in his career. He felt that he personally would have done better following a specialist in a hospital or another academic setting. "They would have had more teaching experience and understood that there was still much we as students didn't know." With respect to nonmedical extracurricular activities, Ari taught hockey to young children and also tutored chemistry. "I did it because I enjoyed it," he added, "not because I thought it mattered on my application."

MD AND DO PROGRAMS

There are two basic types of medical training, and practicing doctors may have received either an MD (doctor of medicine) or a DO (doctor of osteopathic medicine) degree. Currently, there are many more allopathic medical schools than osteopathic medical schools in the United States, although the number of osteopathic schools is rising. Allopathic medical schools provide traditional medical training, and students graduate with MD degrees. A student pursuing a DO completes very similar training, but receives additional training in the musculoskeletal system and osteopathic manipulative treatments. According to the American Osteopathic Association's website, doctors of osteopathic medicine focus on preventive health care and approach the patient as a "whole person" instead of only treating specific symptoms. Further information can be obtained by going to the following website: www.osteopathic.org.

INTERVIEW WITH A DEAN

I was fortunate to interview Dr. Stephen Ray Mitchell, dean for medical education at the Georgetown University Medical School in Washington, D.C. He gave me opinions, tips, and information that you may find useful as you go through the process of applying to medical school. These figures and statistics are approximate and relate to the time of the interview.

Dr. Mitchell informed me that Georgetown received about 18 to 20 percent of all the medical school applications in the country and that (at the time of our interview) the most recent figure for the percentage of female matriculating medical students was 52. According to its website, the school of medicine received 11,237 AMCAS applications for the 2008 freshman class. More than 1,110 were interviewed for a class of 194 admitted students. More recently, according to its website, the school of medicine received 14,377 applications for the 2016 freshman class. 1,011 applicants were interviewed for a class of 196. (accessed 7/9/17)

I asked Dr. Mitchell what he looked for in a good candidate. He indicated that although grades are extremely important, they aren't everything. The interview is very important, too. You may be asked questions such as, "Do you have an understanding of the responsibility of a physician?"; "What are the issues facing a doctor today?"; and "What motivates you to want to go into medicine?" He said that extra-curricular activities are important, but some of them should include medical-related activities. "Without spending time in a medical field and having some medical experience, you won't know whether this is the career for you. A good attitude will help, too, and give you an advantage over another applicant with similar grades and experience."

We discussed the importance of doing research on the school to which you are applying in order to see if this would be a good match and if its philosophy is compatible with yours. We then talked about the economic issues facing students. Tuition can be very costly. When we spoke, the recent annual tuition cost at Georgetown was $40,000, without including cost of living. He informed me that upon graduating from institutions in the United States, 15 percent of medical school graduates will have debts over $200,000, and the accumulated debt for most medical graduates averages $135,000. According to the AAMC website (2017), the median debt for medical school graduates was $190,000 in 2016. There are various opportunities available to prospective students. Georgetown offers the Georgetown Experimental Medical Studies (GEMS) program for students who have been disadvantaged in some way. If selected for the program, these students enter one year ahead of the others and are given the tools and the opportunity to enter the medical field. A significant percentage of these students go on to graduate from a medical school. Some serve in underrepresented and underprivileged areas. Later, you will read about Apryl, a medical student in the GEMS program.

COMBINED DEGREE PROGRAMS

If you are interested in two different fields, you can consider applying for a combined degree program, which allows you to graduate with two degrees simultaneously.

For example, combined degree programs include degrees like MD/MBA (a degree in medicine and business), among others. Physicians today need to have management skills and understand the business of medicine as well as the current healthcare system. Another example includes an MD/MPH (a degree in medicine and public health). An MD/PhD program trains one to become a medical scientist, which includes training in both basic research and patient care. These programs are academically challenging, but some advantages include potentially less time expended and cost incurred than pursuing each degree separately, not to mention the acquisition of valuable knowledge in an additional field such as business, science, or public health. This could place you at an advantage in your career, particularly if you decide to pursue activities outside of clinical medicine such as a leadership position, managing a business, or conducting research.

To find a combined degree program, you can search online by visiting the website of the Association of American Medical Colleges (www.aamc.org) or by visiting the individual websites of each specific medical school to which you are considering applying.

For more detailed information about the numerous U.S. and Canadian medical school programs, you can also go to MSAR online.

AN MD/PHD STUDENT TELLS HER STORY

Rebecca Sadun is an MD/PhD student at the Keck School of Medicine at the University of Southern California. She is also the 2008–2009 Director of Student Programming for the American Medical Student Association (AMSA). Rebecca is currently between her third and fourth year of medical school, with only one year left of a program that averages eight years to completion.

I asked what inspired her to choose a medical career. "I had a unique experience at the age of twelve," she said. "There was an epidemic of blindness in Cuba. A medical team was sent to investigate the cause. One of the physician-scientists on the team was my father. The team discovered that most people affected were adult males, making it unlikely to be caused by a virus, which had been what all of the doctors were trying to treat. After further investigation, the blindness was traced to optic nerve damage from cyanide poisoning, associated with bootlegged rum that resulted from a new government policy restricting the purchase of rum. The trace amount of cyanide was particularly toxic to those people deficient in folic acid, which was rampant throughout Cuba because of widespread malnutrition. Once the team became aware of the cause, they were able to stop the spread of blindness in Cuba." Rebecca told me that she accompanied the team back to Cuba for a follow-up visit. "I was with the team of doctors and scientists who spent eighteen hours a day working, trying to help save people's vision. It was inspiring to see how much the doctors cared about patients who didn't even speak their same language."

In high school, she participated in mock trials as extracurricular activities and was an editor for the school paper. During college, she tried everything from literary magazine editing to equestrian competitions to bench research. "I would encourage students to do what excites them rather than what you think you're supposed to do," she said. As far as mentors are concerned, she told me: "At every stage, I've had people I could look up to and strive to be like. It's very important to have people who inspire you and leave you yearning to grow to become more than you are."

Rebecca completed her undergraduate degree at Brown University before she entered the Keck School of Medicine. She has had a longstanding interest in autoimmune diseases, oncology (study of cancer), tumor immunology, and apoptosis (when cells commit suicide), among other things. In addition to her research interests, she was involved in a couple of patient programs at the Keck School of Medicine, including one "aimed at providing psychosocial support to cancer patients." She also helped develop a "patient education project" at her school, the aim of which is to train medical students how to "educate and therein empower their patients."

She told me about the clinical experience that first led to her passion for patient education. "When I began seeing patients," she said, "I had the feeling they were giving me more than I was giving them. I kept a journal of what patients taught me. I learned so much from them, and I remember the first time I gave a gift back. The patient was a poorly controlled diabetic man with an amputated leg. I took a careful history and asked about his diet. 'I don't eat white bread or sugars,' he said. 'Because of my diabetes, I was taught not to have sugared cereals, so instead I eat pancakes with syrup for breakfast.' I realized just how much I could help this person with the simplest of information. This patient's life and health had been devastated because no one had taken the time to make recommendations clear to him. For this patient, in just a few minutes, I could make a difference. That's the first moment I knew I had a responsibility to do more than diagnose and treat, but also to educate and empower my patients."

She also spoke about the challenges she faces as an MD/PhD student. "The PhD requires a big shift in mentality. In medical school, you usually know what the expectations are. In research, no one tells you what you're expected to do, but everyone tells you when you're doing things wrong. Also, MD students have a shared experience throughout medical school, and so MD/PhD students often feel like they get left behind when they enter the PhD years and their MD classmates head off to work in hospitals without them."

I asked Rebecca what the highlights of her training have been. "Those moments when the two things—clinical and research—come together," she said. "I was involved in a research project in which I was supposed to remove the spleens from mice. One control mouse had a spleen that was too large. I performed an autopsy and found a massive gastrointestinal abscess. Being able to recognize that a large spleen meant likely infection and to diagnose the source of that infection prevented the destruction of an important research experiment." We discussed the cost of a medical education and the fact that some students are deterred by this. "I encourage everyone to continue to pursue their passions. There are numerous scholarships and opportunities," she said, "and as scary as debt is, doing what you find meaningful matters much more in the long run than the finances." Resources include www.aspiringdocs.org. For additional resources refer to the chapter on financing your studies (see Chapter 6).

Rebecca parted with this advice: "It's a long pathway to an MD/PhD degree—on average, four years of undergraduate school followed by eight years of an MD/PhD program—but if you do what you find meaningful and fulfilling, you will be able to revel in the process, and the length of the journey doesn't seem to matter when you're having fun."

AMERICAN MEDICAL COLLEGE APPLICATION SERVICE

When it comes to applying to medical school, timeliness is important. Although preparations begin sooner, students usually begin their application process to medical school in the spring of their junior (third) year of college in order to submit their applications by early summer. Because the AMCAS application is very long, you may want to download the worksheet so that you can complete as much as possible offline. Once you have submitted your information online, AMCAS will verify the information and transmit your application to the medical schools you have designated. Admission requirements vary from school to school, as does the deadline for filing an application.

If you are a competitive candidate who is strongly considering a particular medical school, you may apply through the Early Decision Program (EDP). According the Association of American Medical Colleges (AAMC) website, if you do apply through the EDP, you must only apply to one U.S. medical school by the deadline. If you are offered admission to that school, you must accept. If you are not accepted, you will be placed in the regular applicant pool by the school, at which point you can then apply to other schools. There are pros and cons when considering the EDP. If you do get accepted early, you will not need to send out other applications, and you will save much in time and cost. You will also be assured of an acceptance at an earlier date than most applicants. On the other hand, if you are not accepted early, you will have lost some time with respect to your applications to other schools.

The MSAR details each school's specific admission requirements and indicates whether the school participates in the Early Decision Program.

ESSAY AND LETTERS OF RECOMMENDATION

As part of the admissions process, you will also be expected to write an essay, also referred to as a personal statement or personal comments essay. Your essay can be an important factor in determining whether you make the grade or not, especially if your grades and MCAT test scores are average. Use your words wisely to deliver a powerful message, and make your essay personal, honest, and passionate. Keep in mind why you want to go into medical school. What or who has inspired you? Perhaps someone close to you has suffered from a chronic illness, or maybe you were inspired by a physician who made a difference in your life. What do you plan to do with your future? How will you make a positive impact?

You will also need to provide letters of recommendation. Some under-graduate institutions provide a 'committee letter' or a 'letter packet'. Get advice from a school pre-health advisor. Carefully select the people from whom you will request letters. You should request letters of recommendation from mentors, lecturers, or professors who know you well and can write meaningful letters about your personal qualities and attributes. They should be able to attest to your character, work ethic, and interest in pursuing a medical career. Help by providing them with information such as your curriculum vitae, transcripts, and other appropriate material. Strong letters of recommendation can be very helpful, and weak ones may hurt your chances. If you request a letter and you sense hesitation, it's best not to pursue the issue further with that contact.

EXPERIENCES

In your application you will have the opportunity to describe your work-related, volunteer, research, and extracurricular experiences. Keep a record of these activities and dates, as well as what you learned from them.

INTERVIEW WITH AN ASSOCIATE DEAN

According to Dr. Dawn Cannon, associate dean for student affairs and admission at Howard University College of Medicine, as an applicant you should remember that everyone you meet is possibly interviewing you in some way or another. "It may be a formal inter-view that is documented or an informal interview in which a mental impression is formed. You should always conduct yourself in such a way that the impression you make on a potential interviewer will be positive."

Dr. Cannon feels strongly that applicants should do their home-work in terms of learning about the schools to which they are applying before they arrive for their formal interviews. "We want to see that the student is interested enough to have at least looked at Howard's mission, and to see whether it aligns with their beliefs," she said.

On the website of Howard University College of Medicine, it states that its mission includes providing "students of high academic potential with a medical education of exceptional quality" and preparing "physicians and other health care professionals to serve the underserved." It also states that "special attention is directed to teaching and research activities that address healthcare disparities." Dr. Cannon went on to say that people often assume that, because Howard's mission is to serve the medically underserved, most of their graduates go into primary care after graduation. "Although we do encourage students to enter primary care because of the great need," she said, "we are very aware that underserved populations need physicians in all specialties. The most important thing is to enter a specialty where you will be productive, happy, and needed."

As far as the application process is concerned, Howard takes everything into account, including grades, MCAT scores, writing ability, and experience. "Applicants sometimes underestimate the importance of good writing skills. At Howard, we pay attention to the way applicants write their personal essays as well as their writing samples on their MCAT tests." Dr. Cannon pointed out that it is also important for students to demonstrate some experience within the medical profession, such as working in a hospital, clinic, or physician's office. "The training to become a doctor is so long and challenging," she said, "that it is important for students to explore the field as much as they can so they know that medicine is what they want to do."

A physician on another medical school's admissions panel commented on his interview process. "When I interview a student for admission to medical school, I look closely at what kind of person they are," he said. "In order to get to the interview process, the applicant has already proven to be academically qualified, so I want to see what added value they can bring. They have to demonstrate a commitment to medicine. I ask myself whether I would want this person to be my personal physician in the future."

STAY AHEAD OF THE GAME

Keep track of deadlines throughout your application process, and get everything prepared well in advance. Before sending in your application, review it carefully for errors or omissions, and always have it proofread. Keep copies of everything you submit as well as records of any correspondence. Don't take anything for granted because your career and your future may be at stake. As you go through this application process, remember that you are responsible for checking on your application progress. Make sure that you have completed all the requested forms and sent everything in on time.

After reviewing your AMCAS application, interested medical schools will generally send you a supplementary application packet, with a request for additional (secondary) essays and/or other information. If a school is still considering you as a viable candidate after reviewing your complete application, you will likely be asked to come for an interview. Be aware of and prepared for the financial costs involved both in applying to medical schools and traveling for interviews. Apart from the actual travel expenses, you will also have to factor in the cost of food and accommodations.

THE INTERVIEW

If a medical school admissions committee considers you to be a strong candidate, you will most likely be invited to interview with them. Interviews may be conducted in various formats and you may be interviewed by one or more interviewers. For specific information, check AAMC's Medical

School Admission Requirements website and the school website. Although the interview process can be frightening to some students, it is an opportunity to let your interviewers know that you will be an asset to their school by answering basic questions, such as:

- Are there any aspects of the current healthcare system that you would like to change?
- What were your reasons for pursuing a medical career?
- How would you handle a situation in which you disagreed with a colleague about a treatment plan for a mutual patient?
- What are your strengths and your weaknesses?
- What contributions do you feel you could make to the medical field?

These are only a few of the possible questions you may be asked. Interviewers know that applicants are nervous when coming to interview, and they will usually try to put them at ease. If you are prepared and honest, the interview should go well. Interviewers can usually tell when an applicant is trying to be someone other than him- or herself. Do your homework by reading about the school prior to your interview. Dress in a neat, professional manner, and present yourself with confidence and humility, never forgetting the reasons you want to pursue this path. This is a good time to demonstrate your interests and your passion. Interviewers want to assess your character, motivation, level of maturity, professionalism, and ability to make appropriate decisions. They want to feel confident that you have the potential to succeed at their school. Practice your interview skills. This is a competitive field, and if all else is equal, your interview could help decide whether or not you are chosen for admission to that school.

I asked members of admissions panels how important it was for an applicant to have knowledge about the school prior to the interview. They said that it is good to have at least some basic knowledge of the school. In addition, it is very important to demonstrate true interest in attending the particular school. If you apply to an out-of-state school, admissions committee members want to know that you are passionate about your application and that theirs was not simply a school you added to your list as an afterthought.

Sam, the college student, is already quite familiar with the application process ahead of him, and he will apply online through AMCAS. He hasn't given much thought to the interview, as he feels that it is still far down the road, but he is already thinking about whom he could ask for recommendations. "If I have a good relationship with particular lecturers or professors, I make a mental note to consider asking them for letters in the future."

Medical student Ari found the first medical school interview to be a little scary. Thereafter, he felt quite comfortable with the process. Some interviews are done as "blind" interviews, which means the interviewers meet with you prior to seeing your resume. Ari thinks this is preferable because you can really present yourself as you would like to be presented and they are without preconceived ideas of you. "The other way can feel awkward," Ari commented. He says they look at one's resume and ask questions about it, and the interview generally doesn't flow as well. As a candidate, however, you don't have a choice, and often you won't know whether it's a blind interview or not. Luckily, Ari spent a lot of time researching the schools prior to his interviews. He said he also found a website where other students discussed their interview experiences, and he found that to be very helpful.

Once you know what to expect, the interview process is really not that bad. Let's now hear from a director of admissions at Harvard Medical School.

HARVARD MEDICAL SCHOOL

"Harvard wants to train the leaders in medicine," said Joanne McEvoy, director of admissions at Harvard Medical School. "Students do need to be academically talented, but also should be interesting people with a passion for medicine." According to the Harvard website (accessed 7/24/17), applicants are evaluated based on a number of factors, including academic history, essays, MCAT scores, extracurricular activities, and letters of recommendation. All applicants are required to have completed at least three years of college work and earned a baccalaureate degree prior to matriculation. Applicants interested in applying to Harvard Medical School apply through AMCAS. Applicants will be eligible to file the Harvard supplemental application, which is mailed out to them if they designate Harvard on the AMCAS form. Those applicants who are selected for interviews will be notified by January, and acceptance offers will be made from this group thereafter.

When discussing medical school admission, Joanne McEvoy prefers to focus on medical schools in general. "Medical schools, including Harvard, receive far more well-qualified applicants than can be accommodated. It is a good idea to apply to several schools, because even strongly competitive candidates may not be accepted everywhere they apply." Joanne often gets asked by students which college to attend for their undergraduate degrees. Her advice is to find a college campus where you feel most comfortable. "Somebody from a small town may not feel comfortable on a big campus, for example. At a big research university, you may get to work with well-known faculty and researchers; whereas at a small college, the classes are smaller and the professors may get to know you well. If you attend a college where you have a good fit, it will be easier for you to do your best work, and that will show in your application to medical school."

Joanne also told me that it's not necessary for students to major in the sciences. "What admissions committees want to see in a major is that you can focus on an area in depth. If you study what interests you, not only are you likely to do better academic work, but you will enjoy your time in college more. Medical students can come from all types of disciplines as long as they have completed all the premedical course requirements and have some strength in the sciences."

I learned that admissions committees take everything into account when evaluating a student for admission. "One person may have a strong research background, while another may have demonstrated a deep commitment to community service," said Joanne. "One isn't necessarily better than the other. Grades and MCAT test scores are both indicators of how students will do in medical school. Doing well in these areas can make you competitive, but they will not necessarily get you accepted. In the end, admissions committees are looking not only for a great student, but for those qualities that will make you a great doctor—integrity, compassion, and a talent for working with people."

With respect to the essay, she feels it is important, but only one component. "The essay gives us a sense of how students view themselves. Some talk about where they see themselves in the future, and some talk about from where they have come. There is not one great essay, but you can find an essay that 'sinks' somebody—for example, when it is obvious that they have an inaccurate notion of what medicine is about." She also let me know that students are doing themselves a disservice by sending in an essay with sloppy writing that has not been properly proofread.

"It is mandatory for applicants to have had some kind of exposure to a clinical setting. They need to know what it is like to be around sick people and see firsthand the interactions between different kinds of healthcare professionals such as doctors and nurses." Joanne said that other extracurricular experience is important too, but these should not take the place of clinical exposure. If you also have a passion for music, dance, or art, for example, then by all means, spend some time practicing those activities as well. Medical students and future doctors should be well-rounded individuals.

My final question to the director of admissions was whether she had any advice about the dreaded medical school interview for students. "Just do your best, and always be yourself," she said. "If you have done what you love to do in your undergraduate years, when it comes time to interview, you will be able to talk about your interests with enthusiasm and understanding, and you will shine."

HOW TO CHOOSE A MEDICAL SCHOOL

Before deciding on a particular medical school, ask yourself the following questions:

1. Is there a strong focus on academia/research?
2. Is it an in-state or out-of-state school?
3. Is it a private or public school?
4. What electives are offered at the school?
5. Is this school strong in my particular specialty of interest?
6. Will graduating from this medical school place me at an advantage with respect to getting into the residency program of my choice?
7. What are the tuition and other financial costs?
8. How large is the school? What is the average class size?
9. Are scholarship programs available through the school?
10. Is the geographical location favorable? Would I enjoy living in this area? Is it safe? Is it close to family and friends?

These are a few of the questions you should be asking as you consider where to apply. The type of training varies from school to school. Prestige associated with certain schools may be your deciding factor, or it may be location that tips the balance in favor of one school over another. Yet another important consideration is the financial cost, which you should also consider carefully.

Choosing a medical school is an important decision. After all, you will be spending at least four years of your life there, and there is a good chance that it may be longer if you remain there for your residency training. To be safe, apply to a number of schools, including your home state school. You should include schools you consider safer bets—where you are more confident you will be accepted—some that are competitive, and a few that you believe would be a challenge.

Our panel weighed in on what was important to them when choosing a medical school. "Getting in," said Ari. "If you are not going to get into one of the top ten schools in the country, then it really doesn't matter that much." In that case, he believed that it was a good idea to consider an in-state institution because of the significant savings in cost. But for Sam, a third-year college student only now applying, it's mostly about geographic location and other factors such as the quality of the academic staff and the prestige of the school.

In the event that you don't get accepted into medical school initially and still want to pursue a medical career, there are still options available to you. Take another look at your application to figure out how you can improve your credentials. If your MCAT score is not high enough, you may need to put in the effort to raise it. You can also spend time doing additional study (e.g. a postbaccalaureate program) or research, and reapply to medical school later. Some students attend a medical school abroad and return to the United States for postgraduate training and medical practice.

The AAMC recommends that applicants be familiar with the application procedures of each school to which they apply and that they provide accurate and truthful information in their applications. It is also recommended that all documents be submitted in a timely manner. If you make a decision not to attend a medical school from which you have received an acceptance offer, withdraw your application from that school as soon as possible. For more information, visit www.aamc.org.

Avital, the student who was accepted to one of the Ivy League medical schools, attended the University of Maryland, where she received a partial athletic scholarship. "I had two very good mentors in the departments of physiology and neurobiology, one of whom was also my college advisor," she told me. "They were very different people and so gave me different input." Avital also felt that her interviews went very well. "The focus was on my unique experience. They wanted me to talk about the Middle East and growing up in Jerusalem and my work in hospitals with different patients. They are looking for someone who can bring something extra to the table."

We discussed whether or not she had any trepidation about going to medical school. She told me that she was excited, but also a little nervous about the volume of reading material in medical school. "I have a reading disorder, although I have managed to deal with it," said Avital. "Everyone studies in their own way. When I was in high school, my parents sent me to a tutor, and I have developed my personal method of study, using graphs and drawings for example. The most effective method of study for me is recording the lectures and replaying them at home." I then asked if she had any advice for high school or college students. She told me that in college—because she was an A-type personality and also an athlete—she was always competing, mostly against herself. "I didn't leave much room for a social life. Now I believe the healthy way is to find the middle path. I'm going to try to do that in medical school."

One patient encounter stood out in her mind. "In the neurosurgery unit in Israel, there was a Palestinian man brought in from the Gaza Strip after being seriously wounded in a tribal war within Gaza. It was interesting to see that someone, who perhaps under different circumstances would be viewed as an enemy, was brought in and received first-rate care from Israeli doctors. I saw how humane medicine was."

RATING MEDICAL SCHOOLS

The *U.S. News & World Report* ranks the top medical schools. Ratings are interesting and can provide a certain amount of useful information. In general, however, as you review any school ratings, keep in mind that they give only part of the story. The subject of rating schools is quite controversial. For example, there is not as much significance attached to a school rating unless you know which criteria were used in order to rate the school. You really should choose the school that is the best match for you, based on academics, your personality, and personal preference. Before making your decision, get additional inside information from current students, alumni, and faculty if possible. It is also very helpful to visit the school before making a decision. However, the cost of visiting several schools may restrict your ability to visit many, in which case you may want to take a virtual tour of the school on the Internet. Start by visiting each school's website.

You may find statistics including tuition costs, number of applicants, and class size through the AAMC on its website, www.aamc.org.

We have discussed the application process as well as the medical school interview, and received input from students, doctors, a dean, an associate dean, and a director of admissions. You now know what to consider before choosing a medical school, and you have a resource for finding statistics on various schools. In the next chapter, you will get a view of medical school through the eyes of medical students and physicians.

CHAPTER 5

MEDICAL SCHOOL

This chapter includes an overview of medical school, and several medical students and doctors will talk about their own unique and exciting experiences in the following pages.

According to its website, the University of Pennsylvania (previously the College of Philadelphia) was the location of the first medical school in the thirteen colonies. The school was founded in 1765. Since then, a large number of medical schools have been established in the United States, and there have been significant changes in terms of the student body as well as the curriculum. Most medical schools in the United States today offer four-year training programs, but certain medical institutions and some in countries outside of the United States offer six-year programs. These longer programs usually include more time spent on basic sciences. I graduated from a six-year medical school program at the University of Cape Town in South Africa. During those six years, there was an emphasis placed on acquiring strong clinical skills. I found that the additional time was valuable and gave the students more time for practical, hands-on experience. However, there are pros and cons to each option.

OVERVIEW

The typical four-year medical school curriculum in the United States has been comprised of two "preclinical" and two "clinical" years. During the preclinical years, students study a core curriculum that includes subjects such as anatomy and histology. They learn the basic skills of practicing medicine, including how to perform a proper history and physical examination as well as how to communicate with patients, families, and other healthcare providers. The final two years consist of clinical sciences with clinical rotations. Today medical education has changed at a number of schools. There is more emphasis on interactive methods of teaching beyond the standard lecture format. Students also learn to work in teams and may be exposed to real-life medical scenarios earlier. In the third and fourth years students rotate through the basic specialties: internal medicine, pediatrics, family practice, surgery, obstetrics and gynecology, psychiatry and neurology, among others. Rotations in other specialties such as emergency medicine and anesthesiology are sometimes required. In a teaching hospital, medical students work alongside residents and attendings, gradually learning the skills required to practice medicine. In addition, they take part in clinical rounds during which the healthcare team discusses the treatment of their patients.

Students must also spend time in outpatient settings where they have the opportunity to see how medicine is practiced outside of a hospital. There are opportunities to enroll in electives so that they can gain a better understanding of the specialties that interest them. As a medical student, I chose to do an elective in pediatrics at the Georgetown University Medical Center in Washington, D.C., which only reaffirmed my decision to pursue a career in pediatrics.

Before being able to practice medicine, MD physicians must pass the three-step United States Medical Licensing Examination. (USMLE)

Graduating from medical school is an exciting milestone, but learning does not end after medical school. Most doctors continue their educations for several years in the form of postgraduate training (residency), during which they specialize in specific medical areas of interest. Some go even further by completing fellowships in a number of sub-specialties. Medical knowledge is evolving all the time, and doctors need to keep up with the pace. As a pediatrician, I try to stay up to date not only by reading medical books, newsletters, and journals, but also by attending meetings and conferences, and regularly accessing updates electronically. Additionally, I have found my local hospital medical library to be a valuable resource. Librarians can also help students access academic information as well as information and resources pertaining to the application process.

THE MEDICAL STUDENT'S PERSPECTIVE

Second-year medical student Ari Kestler gave the following account of his first two years in medical school when I interviewed him.

Ari found medical school to be very different from college because now he had to "really sit down and focus." In his first year, he sometimes wondered whether he was doing the right thing and why he was learning subjects that didn't seem to have much clinical relevance. By the second year, everything made more sense as he began to understand the pathophysiology of disease and started interacting with patients more often.

He confided in me about how he has sometimes become affected by patients and their illnesses. In particular, he had recently taken a history and done a physical examination on a patient with an HIV infection and found himself feeling sad for a long time after. He was surprised that he would be faced with such ill patients in only his second year of medical school. Ari said that although medical school can be stressful and one has to work really hard, he enjoys taking patient histories and figuring out problems, and he still thinks that he made the right choice. He says that one has to go into medicine for the right reasons and believes that many students either (1) don't know what to expect or (2) go into the field for monetary reasons and are disappointed later. "A medical student should be hard-working and disciplined, a lifelong learner in the pursuit of knowledge," said

Ari. He would recommend that any student considering medicine spend significant time with someone in the field to learn into what exactly they're getting themselves and to understand why they're going into the medical field.

As for his future plans, he is still unsure. He told me that although he enjoys medicine, he wants a life outside of medicine too, which he thought ruled out a career in surgery. Because of his extensive exposure to emergency room medicine, he would probably choose that field if he had to make a decision today. However, it's still early in his career, and things could change.

A FEW HOURS IN THE LIFE OF A MEDICAL STUDENT

I attended a medical teaching conference—something I did regularly when I was a student and continue to do with some frequency. After the lecture I planned to talk to one of the students about his experiences in medical school.

The auditorium was filled with medical students, residents, and attendings intently listening to a presentation of a complicated clinical case concerning a child. The six-year-old patient in question had recently been in the pediatric unit, and her diagnosis had eluded the admitting team, so several specialists were consulted to help unravel the mystery. The team was now challenging the audience. "She had a temperature of 103 degrees and a rash on admission. Her blood pressure was low." The medical students in the audience were venturing possible diagnoses and asking questions: "Rocky Mountain Spotted Fever? Can you describe the rash? How about the labs?"

"Her white blood count was 17,000 with a left shift, and her sedimentation rate (blood test that detects inflammation) was elevated. She also had a low sodium and potassium level. Along with the rash, she had swelling of her hands and feet."

"Was it Kawasaki disease?" the group asked. "Was an ID (infectious disease) consult obtained?" And so the morning "problem conference" proceeded. It was both an exercise of the mind and an intense learning opportunity. It was attended by various specialists who could share their knowledge and vast experience with the students, one of whom was Brian Allison.

Once the conference was over, I could finally sit down to meet with Brian, a third-year medical student who was in the midst of his pediatric rotation at the time. As I spoke to him, I was mindful of the fact that medical students are always busy, and I was grateful that he had a half-hour break for our chat. He told me that in high school he had considered becoming a doctor and had participated in the volunteer first aid squad. "I majored in neuroscience at Emory University, but I hadn't committed myself to medicine yet," he said. "I didn't really know what I wanted to do."

After college Brian took a front desk job at an outpatient radiology center, where he learned what actually goes on in a medical office. "I also learned how to deal with patients and the 'paper' side of things. Later on, I became more involved in patient care, and I learned a lot about radiology by osmosis." Soon after he started working, he made the decision to attend medical school, so he completed his biology requirement and sat for the MCAT exam. "The fact that I worked prior to beginning medical school gave me a more pragmatic view towards problems like healthcare economics. I also found myself thinking about issues such as whether doctors are over-treating patients or running unnecessary tests at times." He then cited the example of the MRI (magnetic resonance imaging) studies, which are very costly and sometimes not warranted in his opinion.

I asked him about his medical school experience so far. "Anatomy was definitely my favorite course," he told me. "I also enjoyed the laboratory exercises because I like hands-on work. The biggest letdown about the clinical portion is that nurses do so much that medical students and physicians have relatively little patient contact. It makes things somewhat impersonal. My class work prepared me for the clinical years in terms of knowledge, but the practical aspects were different from what I expected. You go to see your patients in the morning, after which you do clinical rounds, and then the residents put their patient orders into the computer for the day." He indicated that much of the work is done away from the bedside.

"One of my favorite parts of medical school was in the second year, when we met weekly with a mentor to discuss clinical diagnosis and went through the thought process of how we should approach patients." Brian told me that he read the book *The House of God* by Samuel Shem. "It's amazing," he said. "Despite the changes and improvements over the years, you still see some of that reflected in everyday scenarios, with respect to human nature and how people respond to stressful situations. I see students still getting frustrated when they have patients they can't make better."

He told me that he enjoyed working with the pediatric gastroenterology (GI) patients most. "These patients are usually not very sick but have problems that impact their lives in significant ways," said Brian. "Fortunately, they are usually easily treatable and curable. This is very rewarding because the children feel better and their parents are incredibly relieved."

Conversely, he continued, entering medical students don't always realize that in many cases doctors don't cure diseases as much as manage them over time. "It has taken me some time to come to grips with this and figure out how to enjoy practicing this type of medicine. I'm not completely there yet," he said, "but I've found that 'shooting the breeze' with patients and learning things about them other than their medical problems helps. Even something as simple as asking them where they live seems to help build a connection." He felt that some patients were more grateful for having someone to talk to than for receiving medical care. "I saw this clearly demonstrated in a man with chronic obstructive pulmonary disease. He taught me a lot about how people deal with the way their illness impacts their lives and their relationships. He expressed a desire to get well, but it seemed that all he wanted to do was talk to me about anything other than his condition. I got the impression that despite having a wife and children, nobody at home was listening to him. More than medical care, I think he needed a vacation, even if it was three days in a hospital."

I also wondered about how Brian was coping with the long hours and frequent on-call rotation. "The medical student work week is limited to eighty hours, and the maximum consecutive number of hours they can work is thirty," he said. "Fortunately, we don't usually hit our max; but it does happen, and consequently we have to make concessions in our personal lives." I was reminded that, as a student and resident, I sometimes worked for longer time periods than that. Restrictions were put into place more recently, and for good reason. When students and physicians work for extended periods of time, they are at risk for inability to concentrate, poor decision-making, and even accidents.

I then asked if there was anything he wished he would have known prior to medical school. "I wish I would have had more knowledge about accounting, business, and economics. More and more doctors are getting away from running their own practices, probably because doctors are not great businessmen."

And what were Brian's aspirations now?

"I would like to own a farm, and perhaps practice rural medicine in the future."

You have now had a glimpse into the life of a medical student through the experiences of two students—Ari and Brian—and you will hear from many others throughout this book.

APRYL'S STORY

Apryl Martin, a second-year medical student at Georgetown University School of Medicine, knows firsthand how important it is to be persistent and not to give up on your dream. "If you really want a career in medicine, you have to be motivated and focused on your goal," she said. "Sometimes you have to be creative and think outside of the box. In my case, telling my story to the right people helped."

Apryl is not a typical medical student, entering medical school only after working as a freelance financial advisor. "I majored in journalism," she said, "although I did take the prerequisites for medical school because I always wanted to become a doctor. In my junior year of college, I took the MCAT exam, but became discouraged because I didn't do well. I graduated and went on to work as a freelance financial advisor." She told me that people at work alluded to the parallels between being an advisor and being a doctor. "In both, one is dealing with the most intimate parts of a person's life," she said, "in this case, money. Although I did well and the job taught me about working in a professional environment and dealing with people, I felt uncomfortable and restless because this was not really what I wanted to do."

Apryl told me that she had several people who supported her along the way so that she could pursue her goal. One of those people was her mother, to whom education was very important, and another was a man who later became her husband. "I told him that I wanted to be a doctor, and he was very supportive right from the beginning. I decided that I was going to try, so I quit my job and prepared to retake the MCAT. I signed up for the Kaplan course and attended from 8 a.m. to 4 p.m. every day. Although it was helpful and I was able to increase my score, it was still not high enough competitively. Despite this, I was invited to several interviews, most likely because of my strong personal statement."

Apryl then explained that she had a difficult childhood. "I was brought up by a single mother who raised five children. We were homeless for some time and went through a lot of financial difficulty. But I had a good role model in my mom," she said. "I was also interested in medicine from early on, and one of my uncles used to tell me I was going to be his psychiatrist. In high school, I volunteered at a hospital; and in college, I worked in an emergency room, so I did have exposure to sick patients."

When Apryl didn't get acceptances from the schools after her interviews, she was disheartened, but one of her mentors, a radiology resident, encouraged Apryl to be open-minded and think about alternatives such as post-baccalaureate programs. She discovered a program for underrepresented minorities, the Georgetown Experimental Medical Studies (GEMS) program at Georgetown University. Students in the program spend an intense year taking many of the first-year medical school courses while learning study skills and receiving faculty support. At the end of the year, they can apply to medical school, and fortunately, Apryl was accepted to the GEMS program. "During that year I was so nervous," she said, "because we could get called to present on a topic at any time. At the end of every day, I felt I had to be sufficiently prepared to take an exam on that day's material. It was tiring, but I learned what I needed to do, too. At the end of the year, I qualified for an interview and was formally accepted to the medical school at Georgetown."

Apryl describes what it is like to be a medical student now. "There are so many emotions at once," she said. "There is a tremendous amount of information one is expected to know, but I am excited to finally learn more about diseases that were only mentioned last year." In her first year, she found gross anatomy to be different from what she expected. "It was more difficult than I imagined, and lab was so long," she said. "At first, when we started doing our dissections, parts of the cadavers were covered, and they weren't fleshy, so they didn't seem human; but once the covers were removed, some of them had nail polish, and that was eerie. I thought to myself, 'That could be somebody's grandmother.'" I asked if anyone had fainted during anatomy lab, and she said no, but surprisingly, a couple of students had fainted during patient interviews at the hospital. "It was hot," she said, "and they were nervous because the interviews were done before their peers and instructors."

Now, her second-year courses include pathology, pharmacology, microbiology and immunology, physical diagnosis, evidence-based medicine, ethics, psychiatry, lab work, and a research requirement. "I am enjoying this year, and I can't wait to work in the clinics next year," she said.

She then spoke about the challenges associated with being a commuter student and a wife in medical school. "In my first year, I worked all the time," she said. "I didn't have time to exercise, and I basically neglected myself. I didn't feel good. This year, I have been better at keeping some balance because I've realized how important it is to keep healthy by engaging in physical activity and eating well. I now advise the first-year students to make sure they have some outlet outside of work."

I asked whether or not Apryl felt she had made the correct choice in pursuing a medical career. "I think I definitely made the right decision," she said, "because I took my time. I think it's important to know with 100 percent certainty that you want to be a physician and that you want to help patients. I know of some people who completed medical school and then realized medicine was not for them."

Apryl grew up in difficult circumstances, and she has struggled (and persevered) in order to realize her dream. Today, things are looking so much better. "Finally, I have a mentoring role," she said, "and students are looking up to me." To all of you considering a career in medicine, she says, "If this is really what you want, and if this is what you know you need to do, go for it, and don't let anyone tell you no."

THE MEDICAL STUDENT-PATIENT RELATIONSHIP

Medical students—particularly those in teaching hospitals—are able to develop unique relationships with patients. Although they have not completed their training, they have already acquired a significant amount of medical knowledge. They may also spend more time with the patients than the attending physicians or residents are able. Patients are frequently grateful for the extra time and attention, and many feel comfortable divulging personal information to students. Medical students can use this relationship to elicit comprehensive histories from their patients and will sometimes learn about pertinent facts that may have otherwise been missed by others. It's rewarding for students to know that they have contributed positively to someone's treatment and recovery.

I remember my enthusiasm as a student. My classmates and I were always eager to learn new facts and practice interview techniques and procedures. To me, a few of the more seasoned residents and attendings seemed jaded in comparison, worn out by their stressful work and sleepless nights. However, we were enthusiastic, eager to learn, and idealistic. I hope all of you considering a career in medicine feel that way now and will remain so in the future.

PHYSICIANS' PERSPECTIVES

Dr. Marc Silverberg, a pathologist, spoke about his years in medical school at Yale. "You have to learn so many facts, but no one teaches you what's most essential. You realize that you can't do it all, so you have to learn to prioritize. I knew that everything was important, but I had to choose what to emphasize at the time, knowing I would have more opportunity to review the information later." He went on to say that the curriculum is not as difficult as students might imagine. "The actual material is not very hard to learn," he said. "It's the sheer volume that makes it almost impossible." He told me that he and the other medical students developed their personal techniques for studying as a result. "For many, developing strategies for learning was a fairly new thing in medical school, but it was very important if one wanted to excel."

Dr. Silverberg told me that in the second half of their first year, the students shadowed community physicians in their offices and occasionally did walking rounds in the hospital. However, they began to learn about the physical examination process in other ways early on. "Yale brought in professional patients," he said. "We could learn to perform gynecological and rectal examinations on those patients who were trained to assist medical students. I can't imagine having to do that for the first time on an actual patient."

Dr. Silverberg described how as a medical student one is filled with all kinds of emotions, including fascination and fear. "I fell in love with every rotation," he said. "I wanted to be everything—a pediatric surgeon, a psychiatrist, a cardiologist—but I found pathology to be the 'queen' of specialties. Some doctors go into pathology because they don't want to deal with patients, but I went into pathology because I truly enjoyed it more than anything else. I could see behind the appearance of disease in every patient. My background as a musician and stage performer was helpful because I could 'fake it' and appear confident even when I was not. Being able to think on your feet in all types of situations is a critical skill in medicine." With respect to being both a musician and physician, he went on to say that he strongly believes there is a connection between music and medicine, and those people who excel in abstract thinking seem to do well in both. He even wrote about this connection in his application essay.

He recalled what it was like learning how to perform procedures such as drawing blood. "As a medical student, I remember drawing blood on patients with TTP (thrombotic thrombocytopenic purpura)," said Dr. Silverberg. "Because they have a platelet abnormality and could break out in petechiae (a rash), we were not supposed to tie tourniquets around their arms. That made drawing blood more challenging, and the task fell to the medical students, including me. It was hard to find a vein; the patient had to drape an arm over the side of the bed, and I would search for a hand or wrist vein that was a little thicker and easier to see."

Dr. Silverberg finally left me with a comment and insight for prospective medical students. "The constant thing about medicine is change. Whatever your undergraduate degree may be and whether or not you change careers as I did, admissions committees want to see that you are teachable, that you can adapt and excel. The ability to learn new things is more important than anything."

Dr. Susan Lovich, a pediatrician, agrees with Dr. Silverberg that there is a large amount to learn in medical school and so many facts for medical students to memorize. On the other hand, she found her preclinical years somewhat less challenging than undergraduate college. "Because many of my exams in undergraduate school were open-book, I really had to think hard to come up with the answers. In the preclinical years of medical school, I found I could do well simply by memorizing facts."

She told me that one of her most intense experiences in medical school was dissecting the hands and face of a cadaver in anatomy lab. "That's when it hit me that I was dealing with a real person," she said. "During that time period, the students in my group were on edge, and the tension was thick." She said it was no wonder they didn't let anatomy students start their dissection practice with the hands and face.

Dr. Lovich did enjoy her surgical rotations as a medical student but recalled one particular event that occurred in the operating room. "During my first rotation, which was gynecology," she said, "I was assisting the resident in the operating room. I had scrubbed up according to protocol and had on sterile gloves, ready to help as instructed. In the middle of the procedure, the resident looked at me and said, 'You just touched your face.' Although I had no recollection of touching my face, I had to leave the operating room. My gloves were no longer sterile. Perhaps that was a sign that I wasn't cut out to be a surgeon."

Overall, however, Susan found medical school to be an exciting time. As a student, she did a two-month fellowship in human rights and traveled to Peru where she worked with a local nonprofit, nongovernmental organization. "We tried to improve conditions in that area," she said. "For students who are interested, international rotations are available in several schools, although medical students may have to pay their own way."

Dr. Lovich mentioned that she learned more than just her curriculum in medical school. "I learned how to deal with people," she said. "I found out that when patients and their families become upset, they may take their frustration out on the medical students—perhaps because they are most vulnerable." She then gave me one example of this situation. "As a student, I helped to care for a patient with a chronic illness," she said. "She needed a surgical procedure, which I attended. One day after the patient's surgery, I was percussing (tapping) her abdomen, and this hurt her; she became very angry at me. I was terribly upset, but the surgeon reassured me. He said, 'She's not angry at you, she's angry at me because I can't save her.' From that experience, I learned not to take things so personally."

Dr. Lovich also believes that medical school teaches social skills. She explained that she can be shy when dealing with people, but she does not feel that way when interacting with patients and their families. "I enjoy patient care," she said, "and feel very comfortable in my defined role as a doctor."

LOOKING BACK—MY OWN MEDICAL SCHOOL EXPERIENCE

I have had so many interesting and exciting experiences throughout my medical career—some wonderful, and others more challenging—and I would like to share a few of these with you now.

Once the excitement of getting into medical school died down, the reality of hard work set in. There was so much to learn and so much to lose if our class didn't make the grade. The fear of failure or disappointing someone gnawed at us. On the wall in the corridor of the anatomy building was a public board on which was posted the results of our recent exams, but only those who passed the exams were listed. I was terrified that I would not see my name, so I asked Cynthia, a fellow medical student, to check the list for me. When she assured me I had passed, I sighed with relief. For that and many other reasons, we worked hard in medical school. While my friends in other fields were up late having fun, I was reviewing organic chemistry or memorizing anatomy—the bones in the wrist and hand, the carpals and metacarpals— night after night.

Once, I brought a skeleton named Harry, which a teaching hospital had loaned me in order to review for anatomy class, back to my grandmother's apartment, where I had occupied her spare room for the last year. At home, I sprawled

Harry out on my bed, covered with the finest sheets and a soft duvet, and I knew my grandmother would not be happy to see him there. Her apartment over-looked the Atlantic Ocean and was decorated with beautiful furniture imported from Italy, and then there was Harry, ruining the *fung shui*. Eventually, I would pass Harry along to a colleague, but using him then to study, I started with the skull and worked my way down, trying to memorize what I had learned in class: the collarbones (clavicles), and the breastbone (sternum), which ended in the xiphoid process. I worked my way down the spine, memorizing the C1 vertebra (atlas), the C2 vertebra (axis), then the C3-7 vertebrae (cervical spine), next the thoracic, the lumbar spine, and finally the sacrum.

Satisfied with the spine, I turned to the arm: the upper arm bone (humerus) and the two lower arm bones (radius and ulna). I knew someone who had suffered a radial fracture after a fall, so I knew that I wouldn't forget radius. Lastly, I reviewed the bones of the leg: the large femur, the kneecap (patella), then the lower leg bones, including the tibia and the fibula. When I was done, I left the skeleton lying on the bed. Though my grandmother was none too pleased, my friends were quite amused when they saw it.

Studying by reviewing clinical problems became a habit. "A three-year-old boy has a history of weight loss and lethargy. His single mother barely makes enough money to put food on the table for her four children. The young boy has a swollen abdomen and is irritable. What's the diagnosis?" asked Mike, a fellow student.

"Kwashiorkor—protein energy malnutrition," several students shouted.

"You are called to see a two-year-old boy who is breathing rapidly and whose cough sounds like a seal's bark," he continued.

"Croup, of course," interrupted Keith.

"At what angle should you assess the jugular venous pressure?" a question to which we shouted, "Forty-five degrees!"

A group of students would meet regularly at one of our houses to study together and test each other's knowledge just like this. The environment was competitive but constructive. We learned from each other and celebrated together when everyone did well.

A Series of Firsts

The bright red blood spurted out as I pierced the radial artery with the butterfly needle, a short needle used for patients with small veins and arteries. After many attempts, this was my first successful arterial "stick." I was proud, as was my mentor, a senior pediatric resident. Someone once pointed out to me that medical school was comprised of a series of firsts—challenges and experiences never before encountered. This is most likely the first time you will start an intravenous line (IV), draw blood, perform an intubation, dissect a human body, deal with the death of a patient, and watch a postmortem examination. Thinking back, viewing postmortems was one of the most difficult aspects of medical school (i.e., exploring the human body after death to determine the cause of death). During these, the students all sat speechless in rows of chairs arranged in circles around the cadaver. We were confronted by a mixture of feelings including curiosity, horror, and fascination. After a while, I think we coped with this by separating ourselves from our emotions. We were medical students now—academicians—not flesh-and-bone human beings with feelings.

Honestly, I enjoyed my surgical rotations. I had been exposed to the operating room before—that is, if you count the time that my friend's father, a general practitioner, allowed me to watch a minor operation in a small-town hospital when I was in high school, or when I had my tonsils out at age two. Those experiences, however, were nothing compared to "scrubbing up" and actually assisting with an appendectomy for the first time. Medical students in South Africa received a significant amount of hands-on experience. In fact, a popular saying among the surgery attendants there was, "See one, do one, teach one," which meant to watch an operation being done, do one under supervision, and then be ready to teach the procedure. This may have been a slight exaggeration, but nonetheless, we did get to perform surgical procedures even as medical students, which thrilled and scared us at the same time.

For example, one day, after following the procedure for scrubbing my hands and putting on my gown, mask, gloves, and booties, I entered the operating room for observation. I remember how tall the Scottish surgeon was and how all of his assistants, including me, had to stand on little benches to reach his height level. I watched him in awe as he confidently cut into the patient's right lower abdomen and pried open the fascia and the muscle. At that point, I felt dizzy, and I was concentrating so hard on not fainting that most of the procedure became a blur. The next words I heard were, "Who wants to close up?" A senior medical student volunteered and deftly closed the surgical wound with sutures. Then, it was all over. "Good job everybody," said Dr. MacNeil, as he thanked us and moved on to his next case. "Maybe one day I'll be able to do that," I thought to myself, and sure enough, not many appendectomies later, I was the student "closing up."

As medical students, one of the highlights was going on hospital clinical rounds. Our group, led by the attending, went from one patient's bed to the next, discussing each "case" in turn. The attending would pick up the patient's chart and recite a brief summary such as, "fifty-five-year-old woman, status: post-cholecystectomy (gall bladder removal)." He would then demonstrate how to examine the patient—for example, how to assess abdominal pain and tenderness while checking for signs of infection. In some patients, when the diagnosis wasn't clear to us, he would ask us to come up with a differential diagnosis. We were very excited to see and examine real patients. To some extent, however, I also felt uncomfortable discussing a patient's personal history, diagnosis, and treatment in her presence.

One of the most rewarding events in the history of one's medical career is delivering a baby. As medical students in South Africa, we had the opportunity to deliver many. During one of our rotations, we spent several weeks living in a maternity home, caring for pregnant patients and delivering babies night and day. We took care of women with postpartum hemorrhage, women with twins and breech deliveries, and babies born with fractured clavicles. Paradoxically, it was one of the most difficult times as well as the happiest in my life. The nurses were in charge of the medical students during that stage of our careers; it seemed as if they could boss us around as much as they wished until we obtained our MD degrees. We students monitored patients' contractions, kept records of their vital signs, mopped up vomit, answered to our attendings, all while regularly being yelled at by Bertha, the short, stout nurse with the bile-colored scrubs, who was aptly named "The Green Vomit."

Those times were difficult also because we didn't sleep—the living quarters were terrible—and we cared for sick patients who often had never received any prenatal care. One time, I assisted with the delivery of a baby to such a woman, and can you imagine our surprise when a second baby emerged? Because she had not had previous access to medical care, she had no idea that she would birth twins. Working so closely with fellow medical students, we formed friendships that would last forever, which made us happy, too. I am still in touch with several of my colleagues from medical school, one of whom gave me a pillow as a gift, a small reminder of our sleepless nights. We also bonded with our patients. I remember how grateful a woman was after I had stayed with her throughout her difficult labor and the delivery of a healthy baby boy.

Studying and working at a teaching hospital in South Africa exposed us students to all types of medicine. Some patients who were lucky enough to have access to Groote Schuur Hospital had the latest in technology made available to them. Still, I couldn't help but notice (and be saddened by) the racial discrimination and how it affected the majority of our patients. For that matter, many patients were in remote areas and did not have the resources to travel to a hospital as needed, so we enacted a mobile clinic comprised of medical students as part of an outreach program. We went into the townships and took medications, infant formula, and needles and syringes for drawing blood with us. For the most part, everything went well on these trips. I enjoyed them and felt like we could at least make a small difference in some remote areas.

LIFE HAPPENS EVEN WHILE YOU'RE IN MEDICAL SCHOOL

Medical school is difficult enough, even if you focus on nothing else. The many hours spent studying and working in the classroom and lab can leave little room for recreational activities and family responsibilities. What happens then when life deals you unexpected difficulties?

As a medical student, one has to be prepared for the reality that everything will not go smoothly all the time. One may have to deal with unexpected illness and friends in need. There will always come family and other social events to attend. Most students have the physical and emotional reserve to handle such occurrences. Sometimes, however, students enter medical school without adequately having dealt with their own health or mental needs. An example may be a student with an eating disorder. The stress of medical school combined with fighting such an illness can take too much of a toll on those particular students. The good news is medical school officials are becoming more aware of these issues and are usually very supportive when students take time off to pursue treatment. They can then return stronger and better able to deal with the complexities of life and medical school. One student told me that she neglected her own health during her first year in medical school. She focused on work to such an extent that she didn't set aside any time to relax. She felt exhausted both mentally and physically. Luckily, before it was too late, she recognized what was happening and restructured her schedule.

Looking back, I certainly remember times when life events made it difficult to stay on the learning track I had planned. The political situation was challenging in South Africa, and many of us wanted to get involved and lend our voices to create positive change. As focused as I was on my studies, I also wanted to remain balanced and see friends and attend family occasions whenever I could. It is good to know that there is life outside medical school.

Although much of medical school is blurred in memory, some episodes stand out clearly. I remember my emergency room rotation and the many trauma victims we treated at a Cape Town city hospital. Stabbings associated with alcohol abuse were all too common. I sutured a head wound of a patient who was so inebriated that he hardly needed anesthesia. My internal medicine and surgery rotations also left a lasting impression on me, partly because of the outstanding teaching faculties. But of all my memories, the ones related to children are most embedded in my mind. I'll never forget the time I went on a home visit to follow up on a child with rheumatic fever. The boy and his parents were so grateful. I still picture the faces of my little patients with malnutrition, measles, rickets, and dehydration so severe that we had to use scalp veins for intravenous access. Even now, I remember their innocence and their hope. Perhaps that's why I chose the field of pediatrics.

Although there were stressful times with many hurdles to overcome, when I look back on my medical school years, I can honestly say they were some of the best years of my life.

CHAPTER 6

FINANCING YOUR STUDIES

The process of obtaining an undergraduate and then a medical degree can be very expensive. Most students are unable to afford these costs without help, and medical students in the United States may accumulate significant debt.

Medical school tuition varies greatly in cost and may exceed $50,000 per year, whereas the annual income for medical residents is relatively low. According to the Association of American Medical Colleges (AAMC) website, for the year 2016–2017, the average cost of tuition for a first-year medical student attending a public school was $30,053 for a resident of the state, whereas the average tuition for a nonresident was $53,399. Tuition will vary greatly depending on whether you attend a private or public school as well as whether or not you attend a school in your home state. Tuition costs are higher for students attending private schools or public schools outside of their home state. The average tuition for private medical schools was $50,599 and $51,880 for a resident and nonresident, respectively. In comparison, four years ago, in the 2012–2013 year, the average cost of tuition for public medical school was $25,979 for a resident and $47,711 for a nonresident, whereas the cost for private school was $44,052 and $45,605 for residents and nonresidents, respectively. The tuition costs above do not include student fees and health insurance, which may be required.

In addition to all of these, there are other expenses to consider. The medical school application process itself is expensive, as are the fees for the MCAT preparation courses and the exam. Some students may be eligible for the AAMC's Fee Assistance Program. See www.aamc.org/fap. You will also have to factor in the cost of books, a computer, and course materials. The amount you spend on living expenses and food can vary considerably depending on whether you live on campus or in an apartment off campus. If you attend medical school outside of your home state, travel expenses can be significant, too.

FINANCIAL AID

If you can't afford the medical school tuition and other costs discussed above, you do have options in terms of financial aid. Most students receive some form of financial aid, most of which is made available through federal, state, school, and community resources. Financial aid may be in the form of gift aid or loans. In addition, some students work while still in school to offset their education expenses.

Gift Aid

Gift aid in the form of scholarships, grants, or awards may be granted on the basis of need, merit, or talent. You may be eligible for need-based financial aid, the amount of which is determined by first assessing what your family can afford to pay toward your tuition and then figuring out your financial needs. It is worth applying for financial aid even if you think that you will not qualify because your family income is too high. An online application for students is available through FAFSA (www.fafsa.ed.gov) free of charge. School deadlines for the application vary, so check the deadlines of your specific schools, and make sure to submit your application on time. Merit aid is awarded on the basis of high academic achievement, and talent awards are made available to students who excel in areas other than academics—music or sports, for example.

Loans

In addition to receiving aid in the form of a "gift," many students also take out loans to help pay for their educations. Unlike gift aid, these education loans will have to be repaid. Subsidized loans, which are need-based, do not accrue interest while you are still attending school, so these are good loans to consider. Unsubsidized loans, on the other hand, do accrue interest while you are in school, so these loans will cost you more to repay in the long run. There are three major categories of loans: student loans, parent loans, and private (or alternative) student loans. Be wary of private loans with variable interest rates, as the rates could skyrocket and place an unexpected financial burden on you later in life.

Work Aid

Students may apply to work in programs run by their school and earn income that can help pay some of their expenses in return. They may operate as tour guides, serve as receptionists, or work in security. Others become resident assistants or work in the bookstore or cafeteria.

Scholarships

There are also numerous scholarship opportunities available to students offered by various foundations, the military, religious organizations, clubs, and other agencies. You may be eligible, for example, if you have a particular talent or meet other specific criteria.

Additionally, several medical schools offer scholarships based on merit.

MAYO CLINIC SCHOOL OF MEDICINE

At the Mayo Clinic School of Medicine tuition scholarships are made available to eligible candidates. According to a school representative in 2017, both merit and need-based scholarships are available. Applicants must apply for financial aid to be considered for a need-based scholarship. As of 2017, the school has three campuses, in Minnesota, Arizona and Florida. For additional information and resources visit www.mayoclinic.org.

Remember that if you do receive outside awards or scholarships, they must be reported to your school's financial aid office. Some students receive aid in exchange for a commitment of service—for example, a commitment to the military. One such example is the Health Professions Scholarship Program (HPSP), a program offered through the U.S. Army, Navy, and Air Force. If eligible and accepted, the military will pay for medical school.

Other Options

If you are not eligible for any of the above (i.e., if you do not qualify for financial aid or a scholarship), you may need to consider a family loan, or private loan. The following websites are valuable resources:

- www.aamc.org
- www.fafsa.ed.gov
- www.finaid.org
- www.fastweb.com
- www.cappex.com

HEALTH PROFESSIONS SCHOLARSHIP PROGRAM

The HPSP offers a medical education in exchange for a commitment of military service. This type of scholarship is offered through the U.S. Army, Navy, and Air Force.

Colonel Stephen Phillips applied to the HPSP in order to pay for school. He spoke to an army recruiter and was offered an army scholarship, which he accepted. He told me that students interested in this type of scholarship can call their local army recruiter or visit the website at www.healthcare.goarmy.com. This program can be investigated and pursued while also applying to medical school. He explained that the scholarship is paid back in time and service rather than money, and he spoke highly of the programs offered. "The army graduate medical education programs are some of the best training programs in the country, and the practice opportunities are good. We are taking care of soldiers and families who are going through sacrifices to serve our country."

I learned that with this four-year scholarship program, one commits to applying for army graduate medical education (residency), and if you are matched with a residency program, you will have to accept that position. Beyond residency, physicians pay back an equivalent number of years. For example, if you took a four-year scholarship, you would pay back four years (in time) to the military after residency training. According to the GoArmy.com website, students must meet the following requirements to qualify for a scholarship. The student must be a United States citizen with a baccalaureate degree from an accredited school and must be enrolled in (or have a letter of acceptance from) an accredited graduate program in the United States or Puerto Rico. The qualifying candidate needs to remain a full-time student during the length of the program and qualify as a commissioned officer in the U.S. Army Reserve. The military will pay for all medical school tuition, college-required health insurance, and books, as well as the cost of most other fees and supplies. Students will also receive a monthly stipend.

You may find additional information about the HPSP through the following resources:

- www.airforce.com
- 1-800-423-USAF (Air Force)
- www.navy.com
- www.healthcare.goarmy.com

INTERNATIONAL STUDENTS

If you are an international student, it may be more difficult to secure financial aid because you will not be eligible for U.S. federal student aid, although you may be able to receive aid from the government of your home country. In addition, some international organizations offer funding to international graduate students. A minority of students may receive funding from medical schools in the United States or from private sources (either in the United States or abroad). The financial aid office can also provide you with information about bank loans available to international students.

FINANCIAL AID ADVICE

As you have learned, financial aid provides students with assistance for their education. Although your family is expected to pay for your education to the extent that they are able, if they don't have sufficient resources, you may be eligible to receive monetary aid.

The following may be helpful resources for financial advice.

Premedical Advisors

Most colleges have premedical advisors to help students with medical school admission requirements and their medical school applications; however, they can also provide valuable information on loans and scholarships as well as other ways of financing your medical education. Sometimes, they refer students to financial aid officers for additional information.

Financial Aid Officers

Financial aid officers at college as well as medical school can give you helpful and free advice. These officers will work with you to develop a plan for financing your medical school education. You do not have to wait until you are accepted into medical school to contact a financial aid officer.

Medical School Admissions Officers

Medical school admissions officers will provide you with information not only about their specific school's admissions policies but also about tuition and other costs, including living expenses. They will probably refer you to a financial aid officer for a more detailed explanation of the options available to you.

Outside Professional Advice

Some students seek financial advice from outside professionals. This is not always necessary, but if you have unusual circumstances and this advice is available to you, it may be reasonable and advantageous to do so.

Whether you receive financial aid or not, you will definitely need to learn to manage your finances and avoid excessive debt. You can find additional resources listed in Part Three.

CHAPTER 7

RESIDENCY

Medical school will provide you with the basic knowledge and training required to be a general doctor. However, to acquire the in-depth knowledge and skill you will need for practicing any particular specialty in medicine, and to become board-certified, you will also need to complete a residency program. Residency consists of three to seven or more years of formal teaching, study, and supervision in a specific area of medicine. While learning and practicing medicine, residents are usually supervised by licensed physicians. Before a physician is able to practice medicine, a license must be obtained to practice in the state or jurisdiction. Doctors can apply for the license after completing the United States Medical Licensing Examination and a minimum amount of graduate medical education (residency). The requirements vary from place to place. The USMLE is a three-step exam, taking at various stages of medical training.

While residents are paid a salary, training is demanding, and they are required to work long hours and be on call many nights and weekends.

THE MATCH PROGRAM

Students usually begin applying to residency programs toward the end of their medical school training via a service, e.g. the Electronic Residency Application Service. (ERAS) Residency programs review each application and may invite an applicant for an interview. After completing interviews, the student ranks his choices and submits a rank-order list to a matching service such as the National Resident Matching Program (The Match). The residency program also submits a list to the same service. A computer matches students to programs based on the submissions, and on a specific day in March, the NRMP results are announced.

Although residency may still be far in your future, I think it's worth having a glimpse into that future. How can you make a good decision about whether or not you want to pursue medical school if you don't have any idea what to expect after those four years of training? Your education does not end after medical school. By the way, although you will be very busy, residency is not all tedious work. In fact, some of my best memories are from those years.

A DAY IN THE LIFE OF A RESIDENT

As a resident on call in a large, inpatient pediatric unit, I was very much in demand. One day, I had only slept for about two hours within thirty-six hours. I had admitted a record number of patients the previous night and was surviving on nervous energy and coffee. After running back and forth from the emergency room (ER) to the pediatric intensive care unit (PICU) and the pediatric ward, answering questions from nurses, medical students, and patients, starting IVs, performing a lumbar puncture, adjusting medication dosages, and drawing blood, I finally managed to sit down to finish my notes. I had barely drawn in my chair when the shrill sound of my beeper went off and made me jump.

Dr. Jones was calling with information about yet another patient being admitted to our floor. "Three-year-old kid, temperature 105.2 degrees, possible sepsis," he said. "Do a full sepsis workup, start him on IV antibiotics, and call me with an update tomorrow. Oh, by the way, his white blood count was 17,000 with a left shift." Before I could hang up the phone, I heard the charge nurse yell, "Dr. Heller, you're wanted in the ER!" My sandwich remained on the table unwrapped.

Much later that evening, after I had checked on all my patients again and sat in on evening sign-out rounds with the students and residents, I went to visit Sarah in the PICU. Sarah, a twelve-year-old girl, had spent many weeks in the intensive care unit and had become well-known to all of us. She affected me deeply, and I was devastated when I learned from Dr. O'Grady, the intensive care attending, that she had very little chance of surviving. Sarah was kind and loving, and sometimes I felt as if it was she who was comforting and reassuring us that everything would be okay. When I reached her bedside that particular evening, she looked pale and didn't greet me as she usually did. I felt disappointed and rejected. It had been a long shift, so I made my way down to the hospital cafeteria for a cup of coffee and sat there for about twenty minutes reflecting on the day. While I was there, I called home to remind myself that there was a life outside of the hospital. Soon, my beeper went off again, and it was time for me to get back to reality and the pediatric floor. A patient's IV needed replacing, so I took care of that; then I went to the resident's lounge hoping for a quiet night. In the lounge sat Rick, a medical student, and the intensivist Dr. O'Grady. Both were silent. I sat down opposite Dr. O'Grady as Rick said quietly, "Sarah died a little while ago."

All of a sudden I was overwhelmed by emotion and began to have doubts about whether I was cut out for this career or not. Was it normal that the death of a patient should have such an effect on me? The attendings always appeared calm under stress and never showed emotion. How would it look if they broke down while placing a broviac catheter or performing a resuscitation or even worse, consoling a parent? I thought of the numerous sick patients I had cared for in the past year and how they had all become a part of me in some way. It was one o'clock in the morning, and I was exhausted. I would feel better the next day, I was sure. We all sat in silence for what felt like a long time, and then I lifted my head to meet the gaze of Dr. O'Grady. A moment before he wiped it away, I saw a tear roll down his cheek.

I was elated when I was asked by the professor and the chairman of pediatrics to do a poster presentation on cystic fibrosis treatments at the International Cystic Fibrosis Congress in Brighton, England. The department would provide financial support, and one patient would accompany the professor and me. The thought of doing a poster presentation wasn't too daunting, especially since it didn't involve lecturing in front of a large audience. It simply involved presenting a poster board with our findings to any interested attendees. The professor was scheduled to give the formal lecture during which time he would elaborate on our research and experience. To my surprise, however, approximately an hour before the lecture, I was hit with the news that I would be the one giving the talk. Although I knew the material well, I was terrified, and I paced up and down the Brighton boardwalk, gathering my composure and formulating my lecture. Much of that day is a blur now, although I understand it went smoothly enough. Only once did I have to direct a question to the professor. It was a scary experience for a resident, but looking back, I would not have traded that day in Brighton for anything. I'll never forget how excited I was to present a talk to such a large audience. My excitement was probably magnified due to the recent breakthrough discovery in locating the cystic fibrosis gene. Although I did not ultimately pursue that field, I felt passionate about the subject, and I gained so much by working closely with patients, assisting in research projects, and learning from outstanding mentors and professors.

RESIDENCY AND RELATIONSHIPS

Because residency training is so demanding, finding the time to devote to a relationship can quickly become another challenge. A greater challenge exists when both partners are residents, which is no longer unusual because of the increase in women pursuing medical careers. In fact, some doctors even marry during residency. Residency is such a busy time that it might make sense to postpone a wedding until after you've completed yours, but I know of residents, including myself, who made marriage during residency work. Although it may sometimes feel as if there's no life outside of residency, one can (and should) find a balance. If you have a partner who is understanding and respects your schedule, you can still have a meaningful relationship.

I ASKED A FEW PHYSICIANS TO DESCRIBE THEIR RESIDENCY EXPERIENCES

"It was the first time I was the one who was able to make important decisions," said Dr. Nelson. "As a medical student, I felt comforted by the fact that I had a resident supervising me. All of a sudden I had to watch over the medical students. At first, I felt insecure, but as time wore on, I became more confident."

Dr. Baynard said: "My life revolved around my work and call schedule. There wasn't much time for anything else. My pager went with me wherever I went. I learned to sleep lightly, always expecting to be awakened, and rarely being disappointed. We didn't get much sleep during residency, but most of us were young, energetic, and passionate about what we were doing, so we survived."

RESIDENCY GUIDELINES

The guidelines for the supervision and work schedules of residents have changed over the years. Today, the level of supervision is much greater than it was in the past, and the system now involves a graduated supervision process, so that residency has become more of a training program. There are also stricter rules with regard to the work hours and the amount of time off between shifts. The Accreditation Council for Graduate Medical Education (ACGME) is the body that is responsible for evaluating and accrediting medical residency programs. According to its website, there were 10,641 ACGME-accredited residency programs in the academic year 2017–2018.

Whatever your specialty, find your passion; then work and learning take on a whole new meaning. Today, with advances in medicine, science, and technology, there are more options for specializing than ever before. In fact, there are over twenty recognized members of the American Board of Medical Specialties (ABMS) and therefore multiple residency options from which to choose.

A good resource is the Fellowship and Residency Electronic Interactive Database Access (FREIDA), which is a directory of residency programs published by the American Medical Association. For more information, visit its website at www.ama-assn.org.

CHAPTER 8

MEDICAL PRACTICE

After graduating from medical school and (for many students) reciting the Hippocratic Oath, one finally becomes a real doctor. With this, however, comes a great deal of responsibility.

THE HIPPOCRATIC OATH

I swear by Apollo the healer, by Aesculapius, by Health and all the powers of healing, and call to witness all the gods and goddesses that I may keep this Oath and Promise to the best of my ability and judgement.

I will pay the same respect to my master in the Science as to my parents and share my life with him and pay all my debts to him. I will regard his sons as my brothers and teach them the Science, if they desire to learn it, without fee or contract. I will hand on precepts, lectures and all other learning to my sons, to those of my master and to those pupils duly apprenticed and sworn, and to none other.

I will use my power to help the sick to the best of my ability and judgement; I will abstain from harming or wronging any man by it.

I will not give a fatal draught to anyone if I am asked, nor will I suggest any such thing. Neither will I give a woman means to procure an abortion.

I will be chaste and religious in my life and in my practice. I will not cut, even for the stone, but I will leave such procedures to the practitioners of that craft.

Whenever I go into a house, I will go to help the sick and never with the intention of doing harm or injury. I will not abuse my position to indulge in sexual contacts with the bodies of women or of men, whether they be freemen or slaves.

Whatever I see or hear, professionally or privately, which ought not to be divulged, I will keep secret and tell no one.

If, therefore, I observe this Oath and do not violate it, may I prosper both in my life and in my profession, earning good repute among all men for all time. If I transgress and forswear this Oath, may my lot be otherwise.

*(J. Chadwick and N. Mann (transl.), **The Medical Works of Hippocrates** [Oxford, Blackwell, 1950], 67) qtd. in **The Cambridge Illustrated History of Medicine** (1996), edited by Roy Porter (p.59) Trumpington Street, Cambridge: Cambridge University Press*

Binding Oath or Dispensable Ritual

I still get chills when I think of the day that I stood with my fellow medical students reciting the Hippocratic Oath, symbolizing our transformation into real doctors. "The Hippocratic Oath is an ancient Greek document," a document dating back to approximately 400 BC, said Stephen H. Miles in *The Hippocratic Oath and the Ethics of Medicine.* It was named after the famous Greek physician, Hippocrates, although its original author is still unknown. The Oath seems to have been written for doctors to guide them in the just and ethical practice of medicine. Today, in the United States, the Oath is taken by the majority of graduating medical students (although most schools use a newer, adapted version).

The Oath speaks to many issues including morals and confidentiality. It also refers to abortion being forbidden, although the same language does not appear in the modified versions used by many schools now. Abortion is a sensitive and controversial issue, and medical schools vary considerably with respect to their teachings about abortion.

Because there have been several translations and interpretations, the exact words and meaning of the original Oath are subject to debate. The value and content of the Oath has also been argued. We live in very different times now, so there are many who do not believe that the same principles and rules are still relevant. Although I think that modifications are necessary, I personally am of the belief that the Oath is rich with ethical principles and ideals that can still be applied to the practice of medicine today. Doctors should always have an ethical responsibility to conduct themselves in an honorable and professional manner, the well-being of their patients at the forefront.

BEING A PHYSICIAN

I have spent a great deal of time thinking about my patients. For me, practicing medicine was never a nine-to-five job. I couldn't step out of the office at a particular time and then automatically forget the day's events. I worried about the boy who had high fever without a known cause, and I hoped that the young girl who was purging (vomiting) had normal electrolytes. I felt frustrated that the twenty-year-old patient with diabetes mellitus was not compliant with her insulin regime, and it saddened me to know that this could increase her risk of blindness, among other things.

As a physician, it's easy to become caught up in the routine of work and treating patients and doing what you know you have to do. Sometimes, when you stop to think about everything you do as a doctor, it can seem overwhelming. When I began to feel this way, I reminded myself that there's only so much I can do and that I can't control every situation. All we can ask of ourselves, as physicians, is to do the very best that we can.

MEDICINE—ART, SCIENCE, OR BUSINESS?

For those of us who began practicing medicine before the 1990s, it is clear that the healthcare system of today is very different than the one when we graduated. A few decades ago, doctors had to rely heavily on clinical skills in order to make a diagnosis, and frequently, the only confirmation that they were right was a positive outcome and a recovered patient.

Today, with sophisticated equipment so readily available, the practice of medicine has changed. Lab results can be ready in minutes, and a patient with pneumonia can have his diagnosis confirmed before he leaves an urgent care center or other healthcare facility. In the United States, we now have medical facilities that are among the best in the world.

Because of advances and developments in newer diagnostic studies, we now have the ability to accurately diagnose many more diseases than in the past. Although a visit to a healthcare facility can become very costly—in part due to an increase in diagnostic testing—this has undoubtedly improved and saved lives.

The Business of Medicine

To a large extent, health care has become a business. A detailed discussion of managed care and business is beyond the scope of this book; however, it would be unfair to write a book for prospective medical students without touching on these subjects.

A few decades ago, it wasn't unusual for doctors to provide courtesy services for a patient who couldn't afford treatment (or even for the neighborhood teachers, clergy, close friends, or colleagues). Then insurance companies stepped in. While in the past it was really left up to physicians to decide on the charges for their services, today insurance companies dictate how much contracting physicians will be reimbursed for their services and general procedures. In some cases, healthcare providers can barely break even. Many doctors feel obligated to contract with these insurance companies in order to remain viable or competitive, especially since patients frequently seek treatment from physicians "in their plan" rather than the best physicians or referrals from other satisfied patients. However, working with insurance companies has led many doctors to huge burdens such as increased paperwork, expenditure of time, and potential financial loss.

DEALING WITH INSURANCE COMPANIES

I'll tell you about one frustrating experience. I called an insurance company on the request of my patient, who was trying to get reimbursed for several of her medical visits. Payment had been denied for reasons not understood by the patient. Apparently, the company had asked me to provide more information about our center because we were out of state. We did not contract with this insurer, but I made the call in the hopes of helping to expedite the deserved refund to the patient. After a long period of time, during which I was instructed to key in my tax identification number and then key in several digits as I was forwarded from one area to another, I finally reached a live person. "Could you please hold?" she asked, and I heard a click before I could respond. "Oh, don't let me be cut off. It took so long to reach someone," I thought as I pictured my patients sitting in the waiting room. Thankfully, after several minutes, the person on the other side returned, and without listening to me first, she proceeded to ask a series of questions: What is your name? What is your callback number? (Why do they ask this? I have never been called back if disconnected.) What is your tax ID number? Your NPI (National Provider Identifier)? What is the patient's name, date of birth, identification number? Claim number? What are the dates of service? I answered every question with as much patience and grace as I could muster. She still didn't know why I was calling. Finally, I was able to ask why the patient's claim had been denied.

"Oh, we don't have a record of that claim," I was told. "The patient must have sent it to her local branch. There's nothing we can do."

"Could you give me the phone number of that branch?" I asked, but was told that they didn't have the number. I checked back with the patient who had indeed sent in the claim to the place I had contacted and had a written denial letter from them proving that they had received the claim.

A few days later, I placed a second call. After surviving the rerouting and initial series of questions, I reached a person who seemed very pleasant. I told her the problem and explained I had a copy of the claim denial, which clearly indicated that their office should have a record of the claim. "Sorry, you'll have to call back. Our computer system is not working," she told me, as I almost dropped the receiver in disbelief.

"I am a doctor trying to see patients. This is taking far too much time," I explained, but was told there was nothing she could do. I was frustrated that nothing had been accomplished, and the following day, I thought I would call one last time.

Again, I had to answer all the same questions. I asked whether the answers didn't register from the first time, and I was told that every call had to be dealt with as a new phone encounter. Finally, I was told that she had found the information and had access to the claims on the specified dates of service. "The claims have been denied," she told me.

"I know that," I said. "I was asked to call to provide more information, which I have now done. Could you tell me why they have been denied?"

"I can't tell you why," she said. "That's what it says on the screen."

"But there should be a reason," I continued. "Could you find out what the reason may be?"

"There is no reason given," she said. I insisted she put her supervisor on the line and she mumbled that she would get him, but no one ever came to the phone.

Even if doctors choose not to work with insurance companies, the paperwork can still be time-consuming. In order to help patients get reimbursed for out-of-pocket medical expenses, even nonparticipating physicians are frequently requested to fill out treatment plan forms that include the patient's diagnosis and the recommended treatment plan. Unfortunately, this does not guarantee coverage for the patient. There have been numerous cases in which patients are denied coverage for treatment that is desperately needed. Examples include patients with eating disorders as well as those with obesity, which was not always recognized as a medical disease. I have heard of situations in which patients had to leave residential treatment centers and inpatient programs prematurely because their insurance benefits ran out, although I am happy to say that this now is beginning to change for the better.

Business creeps into every aspect of health care. A doctor running his own practice has to be concerned with collecting payments and bringing in enough income to cover salaries, rent, equipment costs, malpractice insurance, and other expenses. Physician scientists need to secure grants to pay for their research. All doctors need to be aware of the financial issues that concern their patients. Too many patients in this country are uninsured and may have difficulty paying for healthcare services. Many do not have easy access to health care. The way doctors order prescription medications has financial implications for their patients, too. The same medication in generic form may be significantly cheaper than the brand name medication. Laboratory tests and other diagnostic studies such as X rays, ultrasounds, CT scans and MRIs can be very costly, especially when not obtained within a patient's insurance plan.

My parents and my brother pursued business careers, but I chose a different path. Entering the medical field, I had no idea that I would spend so much time dealing with business issues and negotiating with insurance companies. This was not what I had chosen to do, but I had to learn quickly and develop new skills. There are, of course, medical careers in which one has less exposure to the business side of medicine. For example, if you are a physician in academic medicine or working as part of a group in a hospital setting and don't own your own practice, you will probably never have to deal with many of these issues. You will, however, still need to understand and remain up-to-date with the recommended procedural and diagnostic coding regulations, as well as retain some business knowledge in order to remain viable and competitive in this field.

Unlike other professions, medicine involves a balance of science, art, and business. No physician can fully escape the business side of medicine, although the extent to which you will need to get involved in business will vary depending upon the setting in which you practice.

In the next section, you will read about medicine and ethics. I interviewed a doctor who gave examples of the ethical dilemmas he has encountered in practice, and I will present you with additional scenarios.

MEDICAL ETHICS

"Let me tell you the stories of two babies to illustrate the ethical issues involved in neonatal medicine," said neonatologist Dr. Siva Subramanian. "About twenty years ago, I took care of a twenty-seven-week gestation infant who weighed less than 1,000 grams. The baby was very sick with severe respiratory distress syndrome," he continued. "We did not have Surfactant available to us at the time, and ventilators were not well mechanized for babies. The baby's head ultrasound revealed severe bleeds, and we thought that his prognosis was poor. The baby was slowly being weaned off the ventilator, and I called the parents in for a meeting to discuss whether or not we should continue to provide life support. I explained that their baby would get better as far as his respiratory system was concerned, but that there would be other severe complications. The parents were divided, with the father ready to let go but the mother not. Two days later, the mother was ready to stop life support, but it was too late as her baby had been weaned off the respirator and extubated (tube taken out) that morning. Soon after, he was discharged home." Dr. Subramanian told me that three years later the mother called to schedule an appointment with him. "She brought in a three-year-old child," he said, "sitting in a car seat because he was neurologically devastated. I felt her terrible pain. This had resulted in her divorce, and she was now a single mother. She said, 'Dr. Siva, you should have turned the machines off. If one baby is going to become like this, you should not even try to save others!' That had a powerful impact on me," said Dr. Subramanian. "How could I not intervene with all those other babies when some had a chance of a good outcome? But I realized too that in addition to serving the best interests of the baby, we have to look at the whole picture."

"In the late 1970s, I took care of another very ill 1,000 gram baby," he said. "This baby was also on a ventilator, and for many weeks, we worked hard to try to save him. After more than three months, he was finally discharged from the hospital, and some time after, the family returned to their home overseas. Twenty years later, I received a call from the mother. The minute she mentioned her name, I knew who the baby was. When I asked how he was doing, she couldn't believe that I remembered them twenty years later. She told me that her son had finished high school and was entering a prestigious university as a math honors undergraduate. She had called because he wanted to visit the United States and see where he had been born." Dr. Subramanian told me that the reunion did take place. "The boy was 6 feet 2 inches tall and very handsome. It was wonderful to see him again after twenty years," he told me. "Perhaps we were pushing the envelope when we tried to save him, but sometimes pushing the envelope is the only way to know where the margins are."

Doctors are constantly faced with situations in which they have to make difficult decisions. Consider the following scenarios. Although you are not expected to know how to handle these situations at this stage, they illustrate additional moral and ethical dilemmas you may be faced with when you become a doctor. How physicians deal with these depends on their own judgment, state and other laws, as well as the circumstances pertaining to each specific case.

- Imagine yourself as a practicing physician. You have completed at least ten years of study, including residency. You have learned about the doctor-patient relationship, judgment, professionalism, and responsibility. Your family and friends are very proud to have a doctor in their midst. Your friends find it convenient to have someone they can ask for a curbside medical opinion. You have barely begun prescribing medications to your own patients when you receive a phone call from a neighbor—one who is not a patient—asking you to prescribe a sedative for an upcoming flight abroad. There is a small part of you that feels flattered, but you have learned that treatment should only be provided when a doctor-patient relationship has been established, and as a result, you say so. The neighbor persists, saying that he was unable to see his physician prior to his trip and this would only be a one-time prescription for a mild sedative. He has taken this medication several times in the past and is unable to fly without it. You begin to feel uncomfortable. What would you do next? Would your response be different if he asked for an antibiotic? How about a prescription cream?

- Now imagine yourself as a pediatrician taking care of a young infant. The infant is due for her first set of vaccinations. You know that these vaccinations save lives. The parents refuse the shots due to their religious beliefs. You explain the risks to them but to no avail. How would you handle this?

- You see a sixteen-year-old girl in your clinic. She is crying uncontrollably and soon confides to you that she is pregnant. You encourage her to speak to her parents, but she refuses, explaining that she is afraid of what her father would do if he found out. She then says that she has made up her mind and she wants an abortion. How do you proceed?

- You are the internist of a twenty-one-year-old woman who has anorexia nervosa and has rapidly lost a significant amount of weight. You examine her and recognize that she is in danger medically and needs to be treated in a hospital. You advise her to go to the nearest hospital for an evaluation and inform her that you will make the necessary arrangements for her admission. She refuses hospitalization. How would you react, and what would you do next?

These are only a few of the types of ethical issues doctors face all the time. Practicing medicine will require you to have a good knowledge of the law and strong personal, moral, and ethical codes. For example, states vary on a number of laws—particularly those regarding minors, such as consent to contraception and abortion—so you will need to become familiar with the laws in the state in which you practice. You will also encounter situations in which you need to make difficult decisions that go beyond legal obligations and are instead based on ethical and moral principles.

UNDERSTANDING CULTURAL, SOCIOECONOMIC, AND RELIGIOUS INFLUENCES

"What could that be?" The medical student looked at me for an answer, but I, a young resident at the time, could only stare back at her equally perplexed. We were in the midst of our weekly rotation in an outpatient clinic in Northern Virginia. The infant lying on the examining table appeared to have an unusual skin condition. His skin felt prickly, his hair almost needle-like. Otherwise, he was active, crying appropriately, and neither of his parents seemed the least bit concerned. They had brought him in for his routine checkup. It was only after several questions (and then finally the right one) when the student and I reached a diagnosis—honey! The parents reported that in their particular culture it was quite acceptable to cover their babies in honey. Mystery solved.

In South Africa, we were exposed to patients from various cultural backgrounds. All physicians need to be aware of the cultural diversity in the United States. In whatever setting you decide to practice, you must be knowledgeable about your patient's frame of reference in order to provide appropriate treatment effectively.

Ignorance on the part of a provider can lead to inadequate treatment. The following scenario is one example. A healthcare provider spent a long time with a patient and his family. The patient was morbidly obese and was encouraged to lose weight. The provider gave the family advice on nutrition, emphasizing the importance of eating more fresh fruits and vegetables. She also recommended that the patient become more physically active by going for walks or joining a gym. When the patient returned two weeks later, the healthcare provider was surprised that he had not lost any weight. She asked about his fruit and vegetable intake and about his physical activity. Embarrassed, the family admitted that they had not made any changes. They could not afford to buy fresh fruits and vegetables or join a gym, and because of their unsafe neighborhood, walking outside after school was not an option.

Although well intentioned, the healthcare provider had not taken into account the family's life circumstances, and therefore, she couldn't provide optimal treatment in this case.

Miscommunication leads to errors. A physician told me how she almost made a mistake because she didn't fully understand her patient's father. "A child came in with a cough," she said. "I listened to his chest and heard a few wheezes. I asked the father what medicine they had given him, and I thought he said Advair. Because I had heard wheezing, I jumped to a diagnostic conclusion and asked if his son had asthma, which was sometimes treated with Advair. The father explained that he did not have asthma, and the medication was given for fever. It turned out to be Advil, but because of his accent, I heard it as 'Advair.' That taught me to be cautious about making assumptions." Essentially, it's good to double-check whenever there is room for doubt.

A significant percentage of the population speaks a language other than English at home. According to the U.S. Census Bureau, (2009–2013 data) almost 80 percent of the population five years and older speak only English at home, but the percentage of the population that speaks English less than very well is reported as 8.6 percent.

Ignorance about cultural beliefs has led to healthcare disparities and can result in negative outcomes. Because of cultural differences and language barriers, doctors may not fully understand patients and their medical histories. This may lead to inadequate or unnecessary testing as well as different, inappropriate treatments. Of course, patients may not always understand their doctors and cannot therefore follow their advice. If healthcare providers are not aware that patients may be using herbal or other traditional treatments, additional medications can lead to problematic drug interactions. Disparity in treatment can also occur because of biases or stereotyping on the part of the healthcare provider. Educating medical students about cultural diversity can reduce these problems.

Dr. Susan Lovich has taught students about cultural diversity and health disparities. She said that it is very important for medical students to know their own biases. They need to be aware of any preconceived ideas and stereotypes they themselves may have, so they can compensate in their field. "It is more difficult and sometimes frustrating to deal with families when there is a cultural or language barrier," she said, "but you must treat people as you would want to be treated. That may involve putting in extra effort. In the case of language barriers, it means having access to interpreters or language lines."

Another piece of advice she gave for medical students and residents is to become familiar with the demographics of the area in which they plan to practice. "I helped create a curriculum for residents going abroad to provide medical care," said Dr. Lovich. "Before the residents traveled to Honduras, we required them to research the background and culture as well as the diseases that were more common in that population." Because of the frequency of international travel today, it has become more important for medical students and doctors to be aware of diseases seen all over the world.

It is helpful (if not essential) to understand the belief systems of different cultures. Dr. Lovich gave an example. "In certain cultures, the father is seen as the head of the family," she said. "If he does not speak English, you may find a situation in which the patient—a child—is doing the translating. It changes the balance of power. It falls upon you to figure out what the patient's perspective is. Also, religion may play a crucial role in treatment. For example, Orthodox Jewish families don't drive on Saturdays, so doctors need to take this into account when making a treatment plan."

Patients come from all types of cultural and socioeconomic backgrounds. They also differ with respect to religious and moral beliefs. Many religious groups differ in their views on contraception, abortion, end-of-life care, not to mention the responsibilities of males and females, parents, children, and grandparents. Learning about human diversity is among the great rewards and responsibilities of being a doctor.

THE MEDICALLY INFORMED PATIENT

"I think I have bipolar disorder," a teenage patient once told me. "I heard about a medication on a television commercial. Could that help me?"

"Can you prescribe this antibiotic for my child's cough?" asked a father of a one-year-old infant.

"I don't agree with the diagnosis my dermatologist made," a young girl told me after consulting with a specialist. "I checked my symptoms on the Internet, and it didn't fit."

These are the types of questions and statements you may hear from patients and parents. In the past, it was usual for patients to refer to their doctors as the ultimate authorities when it came to their mental and physical health. Doctors were highly regarded and respected, and their judgment was rarely questioned by patients, but today, that is not always the case.

Many patients and their families feel quite comfortable questioning and even challenging their doctors. Patients today have ready access to online medical data on a vast array of topics. Once they enter a doctor's office, they have frequently done some preliminary research, which may or may not be accurate. The challenge is to sort out information from misinformation and explain any discrepancies. Doctors need to involve patients in their treatment and formulate plans that are mutually acceptable.

At our outpatient center in Maryland, we ascribed to the philosophy of a team approach to health. The patient is (and should be) a key member of his or her treatment team. The role of current and future doctors is less likely to be authoritarian, but rather cooperative.

We have discussed the significance of cultural, socioeconomic, and religious diversity. The next section will focus on women in medicine.

WOMEN IN MEDICINE

I interviewed two female doctors to get their perspectives on being a woman in the medical field.

"When I was a medical student in South Africa," said Dr. Naomi Baumslag, "I remember one of the male students asking me, 'Naomi, would you make the tea, because you're the girl?' I answered back, 'You don't carry the ECG machine for me, so I don't make your tea.'"

Dr. Baumslag, a physician who also has her master's in public health from Johns Hopkins School of Hygiene and Public Health, said that female physicians in South Africa received significantly lower salaries, were often passed up for leadership positions, and received unequal treatment. "In my third year of medical school," she said, "I received a letter which read: 'Dear Miss Baumslag: If you should fall pregnant, you should expect to stop attending class.'" Dr. Baumslag could not believe what she had read. "In South Africa, I definitely had a lower salary than my male colleagues," she continued. "The attitude was: You have a husband. You shouldn't worry about money, because your husband is earning a salary."

Dr. Baumslag told me that this inequality was still noticeable even after she moved to work in the United States. "When I came to Washington, D.C., I was offered a job at Health and Human Services. I was also interviewed for a position at a well-known academic institute. The chairman looked at my resume and said, 'I see you have a thirteen-year-old daughter. How would you manage?' I was astounded and replied, 'It's none of your business, and there's no way I could work with someone with this attitude.'"

Dr. Baumslag ran several programs, one of which was a family care program at a well-known university in the United States. "The chairman of community medicine offered me a part-time job as an assistant professor at the university," she said. "Although I wanted the job, I knew that I was qualified for a higher position. My brother, who was a professor at another institution, recommended that I ask for a full-time associate professorship instead." Dr. Baumslag was hesitant because she knew that it was uncommon for women to be accepted to those positions; however, she decided to give it a try. "My brother told me exactly what to say, and I wrote it down word for word. When I called the chairman, I was so scared that I read to him exactly what I had written down, and to my surprise, I was accepted." She told me that women have to look at what is being offered to men in similar positions and expect the same compensation. Women still receive lower salaries, and though the gap is closing, there still exists real bias and discrimination.

Another female physician told me that there were only a few women when she attended medical school. "In one rotation, I went way above and beyond what was expected of me," she said. "I gave medical grand rounds as a discussant for a case, and it went very well. Later on, a male physician even asked me how I knew all this information—the implication was that it was unusual for a female to be that knowledgeable. When it was time for me to be graded, I only received a B. I could not figure out why. During my residency training, there were a few patients who would say, 'Hey, cutie,' or call me nurse."

I asked whether she had encountered any discrimination in practice. "I recall one incident that happened when I was working at a university," she said. "I had young children at the time, and because of a problem with the babysitter, I had to be late one day. Luckily, I had no patient responsibilities on that particular day, which was going to be devoted to doing research. Instead of being understanding of my situation, my boss was livid. On a separate day, one of the male physicians called in with car trouble. He was scheduled to perform surgery that day. The boss excused him without question. Thankfully, this type of situation happens less and less today as more women enter the field."

Although the number of women in medical school and in practice has increased dramatically, gender inequality still exists. A large percentage of women enter primary care specialties such as internal medicine, family practice, pediatrics, and obstetrics and gynecology, whereas specialties such as surgery and anesthesiology are still dominated by male physicians.

Incorrect assumptions also exist. On a recent vacation in Florida, I chatted with a couple, and the husband began sharing medical stories with me. (After you graduate from medical school, you will find that as soon as people learn you are a doctor, oddly enough they will divulge the most intimate details of their medical histories.) This man told me he suffered from neuropathy. "I went to see a—not a urologist," he said.

"A neurologist?" I offered.

"Yes, yes," he told me, "and it was so strange. The doctors in the office were a husband-and-wife team, a neurologist and gynecologist. When they asked me who I wanted to see, I said the husband of course, assuming he was the neurologist. I was so surprised when I found out the wife was the neurologist, and he was the gynecologist."

We have heard the views of two female physicians, and we have heard stories of gender inequality. Now, let's discuss what issues female medical students will need to consider.

Considerations for Women

Women do need to take certain factors into consideration before entering the medical field. For one, if they decide to start families, they should know how much maternity leave will be offered. Because they are often the caregivers, those with families will face the challenge of creating balance between their family lives and their careers. Single mothers may struggle to find babysitters, especially at a moment's notice when called into work unexpectedly. Having said this, men may be the primary caregivers and therefore face similar issues. Also, in spite of practicing in the twenty-first century, women may be confronted with prejudice and unequal treatment in certain situations. If they decide to enter a specialty such as surgery, they need to be comfortable working in a field that is still male-dominated. That said, neither women nor men should have to tolerate any form of discrimination.

THE LIFE OF A PEDIATRICIAN—MY OWN INSIGHTS

After graduating from medical school in South Africa, I completed a three-year pediatric residency program at Georgetown University Medical Center in Washington, D.C. I don't think anything quite prepares one for residency, but I'm grateful for having had the experience. There is a steep learning curve during the first year of residency. I remember having to appear confident when I was not. There were times when I had to console patients and families when I needed consoling myself. During that year, we put much faith in our senior (third-year) residents and especially in the chief resident. They were our heroes who seemed to know everything. We tried hard to handle small crises on our own; however, when we felt we truly needed help, we would succumb. We would page the senior residents—sometimes late at night or in the early hours of the morning—and they never let us down.

During my first year in residency, we learned to perform procedures such as intubations, lumbar punctures, suturing wounds, splinting fractures, and arterial punctures. We escorted premature babies on ventilators to tertiary care hospitals in ambulances. We were taught to diagnose illnesses such as meningitis, Kawasaki disease, pleural effusions, Lyme disease, malaria, and achalasia. We were expected to calm worried parents, put patients at ease, give presentations to fellow residents and attendings, assist in the emergency room, take night-call shifts every third night, and deal with stress and a constant lack of sleep.

However, I survived, as we all did, and after residency, I decided to go into private pediatric practice. I was lucky because while I was still a resident, I received a call from a pediatrician in an established group private practice and was asked to spend some time working there with the goal of joining in the future. She recommended that I do further training in the field of adolescent medicine so that I could bring new skills to the group and perhaps assist with starting an adolescent center. I took her advice and spent my electives and free time learning as much as I could about adolescent health. I spent several weeks working with a gynecologist, learning how to evaluate teenagers with sexually transmitted diseases, pregnancy, and even abuse. Following the gynecologist as she saw one patient after another taught me not only about gynecology but also about the physician-patient relationship. I attended conferences whenever I could.

After completing my residency, I was offered a regular position in the pediatric group practice and eventually became a partner. I found many advantages to being part of a group practice, one of which was the excellent support from experienced colleagues with whom I could discuss medical conditions and concerns. In a group practice, although "call" will be busier, there will probably be fewer "on-call" nights and weekends, since call duty can be shared with partners. Going on vacation is more feasible when colleagues—ones who are already familiar with your patients and your treatment style—can take over their care. The cost of liability insurance may be lower per physician than taking out an insurance policy for a solo practice. On the other hand, there are advantages to practicing on your own, especially if you have a strong desire to make all your own decisions and know all your patients well.

I greatly enjoyed fourteen years in private pediatric practice in Northern Virginia. Time passed quickly, and now, as I look back on those years, I am filled with mixed emotions. I remember many of the happy times, like when very sick patients got better or when children I cared for became healthy adults and came back to visit me—sometimes with babies of their own—or when families sent me kind letters. But there were also sad times, such as when a young boy was killed in a car accident and when another boy, following a severe infection, spent many days in the pediatric intensive care unit barely hanging onto life.

Looking back now, I remember how afraid I was on my first day seeing patients in the private practice. It was a large practice, and I was one of several pediatricians. The healthcare team included nurses, laboratory technicians, and a lactation consultant. Everything was so new to me—the office, the procedures, the equipment, and the staff. There was a nurse assigned to work with me for the day. I completed routine physical examinations on my first two patients, an eight-year-old boy and a two-month-old baby girl. Although everything went relatively smoothly, I was sure everyone noticed my insecurity. This felt different from being a medical student or a resident. I was on my own now, and I wasn't sure that I was cut out for this job.

Just then, a twelve-year-old girl named Becky was rushed into our office with a severe asthma attack. Her chest was so "tight" that one could barely hear wheezing or even breath sounds. I pulled out the oxygen and an oxygen saturation monitor, and set up the nebulizer with medication to open up her airways. She breathed in the nebulized mist as her mother held her hand and tried to calm her. After receiving the treatment, Becky was a different girl; she was even able to joke with us. My confidence quickly returned, and from then on, I already felt like I belonged in that pediatric clinic. For the partners, it became our second home. We soon started an adolescent center in which I spent most of my time. It was here that I really became interested in the field I would eventually enter—adolescent eating disorders.

I spent four days each week seeing patients at either one of our two offices, and on the fifth weekday, I would relax or attend meetings or lectures. We rotated night-call among our six doctors, so although call was sometimes grueling—I received fifty calls one day!—there were still moments of respite.

Most of my mornings were spent seeing patients in our walk-in clinic. This time was reserved for patients who were ill and needed to be seen on the same day. They came in with everything, including infections, minor trauma, headaches, vomiting, and even head lice. I was never sure what to expect, and that definitely kept me on my toes and made things interesting. Most of what remained of my day was then spent doing checkups and seeing children with ear infections, upper respiratory infections, and other viruses, but sometimes, we would see patients with uncommon illnesses, like Kawasaki disease, or such acute problems as appendicitis and meningitis. When I wanted a second opinion, I could simply consult one of the five other pediatricians. Occasionally, I had to hospitalize a patient, and eventually, we developed a good rapport with the admissions staff of the local hospital, which greatly facilitated admitting our patients quickly when it became necessary.

On days that I had hospital duty, I set my alarm clock for 5:30 a.m. so that I could start my clinical rounds at 7:00 a.m. (I remember that I had become quite good at dressing in the dark so that I wouldn't wake my husband.) It was at least a forty-five-minute drive to the hospital, so I used the time to listen to tape recordings—either CME (continuing medical education) or music recordings—but the drive passed quickly. Although I was often tired, making hospital rounds was very rewarding because the parents really appreciated pediatricians taking the time to give their children personal attention. It was also wonderful visiting new moms and dads and being able to reassure them that their babies were healthy. Parents have told me that it was a great comfort seeing a familiar doctor instead of the hospital pediatrician or neonatologist on call.

As I went on rounds, I checked in with the pediatric residents who "covered" my patients. They would fill me in on any pertinent information, such as whether there had been any problems overnight or any abnormal laboratory results. Making rounds was never predictable. One day I had to resuscitate a young patient with a tracheostomy tube who had developed respiratory arrest when the tube became blocked. Thankfully, the patient did well. After reviewing each patient's chart, I would write my progress note, and when I was done, I returned to my office to see my scheduled patients. Today, much of the inpatient care has been taken over by hospitalists and residents, and it is no longer routine for pediatricians in private practice to make clinical rounds on their patients in the hospital.

Being on call became a way of life, but it was something I had to learn to live with as a physician. I always felt attached to my beeper and the phone. Even when I slept, I slept lightly, ready to take that emergency call. Patients and families called with all sorts of problems. Some only called for serious emergencies, such as acute abdominal pain or high fever, while others called in the middle of the night with nonurgent questions. In fact, I remember being awakened from sleep at 2:00 one morning by a mother asking me how long she should breastfeed on each side.

I felt happy and comfortable in the practice but was always compelled to learn more. I had a passion for writing, edited a quarterly newsletter for the practice, and later began writing medical books.

I have always been interested in adolescent issues and gradually began studying more in this field, specifically eating disorders. I soon opened a multispecialty center for the treatment of eating disorders and obesity in adolescents. Although there were times when I felt tired and challenged by patients with difficult problems, it was worthwhile. I have become more and more hopeful that with appropriate treatment, patients with eating disorders really can get well and lead happy, meaningful lives.

Someone once asked me what I found most difficult about being a doctor and what my biggest rewards were in the field. For me, one of the toughest parts is carrying such an enormous responsibility for someone else's health and worrying about very ill patients. The other challenges are the irregular hours with little downtime as well as keeping up to date with the vast amount of new information and the major advances in science and medicine. Dealing with insurance companies and large amounts of paperwork can be a nuisance, but one gets used to this. You will need to be prepared for a healthcare environment in which doctors are scrutinized more than ever before. In the past, I have heard doctors faulted for not "telling" on each other when they see a wrongdoing. Prior to the establishment of regulatory medical boards, there were rarely disciplinary actions against doctors. Today, doctors find themselves constantly evaluated by the medical boards, insurance companies, and their peers. Some find themselves caught in a system that does not always seem supportive of doctors.

On the other hand, the rewards are many. Establishing relationships with families, being allowed to share in their experiences, and helping others is very gratifying. I have also found that pursuing other aspects of the medical field such as writing medical books, lecturing to students and colleagues, and publishing articles can keep one motivated, interested, and continuously learning. When I became involved in public health issues—testifying with the goal of improving school lunches and increasing physical activity in schools to help combat childhood obesity, for example—I felt I was making a difference, and I believe that's basically what we as doctors really want to do. A medical career is a mixed blessing; the burden of the responsibility weighs heavily at times, but the positive experiences, the satisfaction of helping others, and the good memories more than make up for the problems. I've had thousands of patient encounters, but some rewarding experiences in particular remain vividly in my mind.

"It's a Miracle"

There are a couple of treatments that can appear miraculous to patients and their families. One of these is the use of oral prednisone (steroids) for the treatment of asthma and allergic reactions such as poison ivy. An example of a second follows.

In my first year of practice, a three-year-old boy named Sammy was carried into our clinic by his father, who was sobbing. "I think I've broken his arm," Mr. Roberts cried. Sammy, who was also crying now, was holding a teddy bear in his right arm, but his left arm was hanging limply by his side. "He won't move it at all," continued his father.

"What happened?" I asked, trying to calm them both, albeit unsuccessfully. Mr. Roberts went on to explain how Sammy had run into the road after a ball and how he had grabbed his son's arm to pull him to safety. Thankfully, his son had been rescued from the street, but he had not moved his left arm since that time.

I recalled reading about "nursemaid's elbow" many times before, and I remembered our emergency room attending teaching us how to perform a series of moves until…"you will hear a click." I had visualized this scenario many times but had not had the opportunity to perform this maneuver, that is until now. "Did your son fall or sustain any other injury to his arm?" I asked Mr. Roberts.

"No, he didn't fall or hit his arm against anything."

"Let's just see," I said. "It's probably not broken. We call this a nurse-maid's elbow."

Then, I took Sammy's arm in mine, holding his left elbow with my left hand and his hand in my right. I gently went through the moves I had been taught. For a split second I wondered if I was doing the right thing, and then all of a sudden, I felt and heard the click! I waited and watched. The crying stopped. Sammy climbed out of his dad's arms and just stood there. I waited a little longer, then took a brightly colored sticker, and offered it to him. To my delight, he dropped his teddy bear and took the sticker with his right hand. I held out a second sticker, and this time, smiling, he reached up with his left hand and took the sticker. All his father could say as he left the clinic room was, "It's a miracle!" What a gratifying feeling that was.

CHAPTER 9

THE FUTURE OF MEDICINE

There have been significant advances and discoveries in the medical field over the past century, but never has there been a time like now, when change is occurring so rapidly with such an explosion of information. Major technological advances, coupled with greater understanding of biochemistry, biology, and neuroscience, have led to the understanding of the causes and treatment of diseases, some of which were deemed untreatable in the not-too-distant past. The widespread use of the Internet and other computer technology has led to greater ease of communication with experts around the world, and given us the ability to access and transfer information rapidly. Today, a clinician in a foreign country can contact physicians and researchers in the United States and access up-to-date information on most medical topics simply by logging on the Internet. We in turn have reciprocal access to data in other countries.

WHAT WILL MEDICINE AND THE HEALTHCARE SYSTEM OF THE UNITED STATES LOOK LIKE IN THE FUTURE?

There are many factors to consider. The U.S. health challenges of today and the future are different from the past in many respects. The population has grown significantly and is now over three hundred million. Americans are living longer, so the population of elderly is large and growing. As a result, we now face a growing shortage of geriatricians and must focus more on caring for the aged. Hospice care and palliative medicine are important innovations.

More attention has been given to prolonging life and the prevention and treatment of the symptoms of aging. But although we have the ability to prolong life, how far do we go? To what degree is it ethical to prolong life if a certain quality of life cannot be preserved?

Advances in Genetics

The field of genetics is fascinating, and greater understanding of this subject has increased our knowledge about numerous diseases including cancers. Located at the terminals of chromosomes are repetitive sequences of DNA known as telomeres, which essentially protect the ends of chromosomes from being destroyed, thereby protecting the DNA strand as a whole. Telomeres, therefore, usually limit the number of times cells in our body can divide. The function of telomeres also appears to have associations with cancer as well as the aging process. Future research on telomeres and aging may lead to further advances in the treatment and prevention of cancers, one of the leading causes of death in the world.

Human genome sequencing and embryonic stem cell research have opened the doors to all sorts of possibilities in the future. This will potentially lead to earlier identification of abnormalities and breakthroughs in the treatment of many diseases. According to Dr. Michael Watson, executive director of the American College of Medical Genetics and adjunct professor of pediatrics at Washington University in St. Louis, only recently have we begun to appreciate the importance of copy number variation, in which large sections of human DNA are replicated or deleted. These variations or changes can be associated with previously undiagnosed diseases, increased susceptibility to diseases, and in some cases, resistance to disease. Examples of disorders with copy number variation include trisomy 21 (Down syndrome), Prader Willi syndrome, and autism, among others. Hopefully, modern technology will allow us to detect these changes more readily.

Genome sequencing will also allow scientists to predict susceptibility to certain diseases in individuals. Although this has obvious positive implications for the prevention and treatment of cancers, diabetes, and heart disease, it also carries with it ethical concerns. "We're at the point where we have to balance what information we need for the common good against protecting the individual's privacy," said Dr. Watson. "Because we don't know how to interpret much of the human genome, we need to be directive about what we test for and what we report out." He said that an enormous amount of money was spent on the human genome project, and we now need to focus on understanding what genes do, what gives us clinical value. "We are now moving more towards translational activities and evidence-based genetic screening," he continued. Dr. Watson then spoke about the progress that has been made in terms of newborn screening as an example. "Whereas in the past babies were only screened for two or three conditions," he said, "today over four million newborns are screened for a large number, including phenylketonuria and hearing loss."

Stem Cell Research

Human stem cells are unspecialized cells that have the ability to renew themselves or proliferate through cell division, with the added potential to develop into different, specialized cell types under certain conditions. Stem cell research offers great hope, including (but not limited to) the potential to treat diseases that currently remain untreatable, as well as the ability to test new drugs in the laboratory.

Diseases of Lifestyle

The fact remains that patients are still dying in large numbers from heart disease and cancer. However, fewer patients suffer from diseases of undernutrition, such as marasmus, scurvy, and kwashiorkor. Instead, people are suffering more from obesity and its complications, accidents, smoking, substance abuse, and other diseases related to lifestyle choices. Obesity has been associated with morbidity—rivaling that of smoking—and because of obesity, more young patients are seen with type 2 diabetes, a condition previously only seen in adults. Every office visit with a patient should be thought of as a chance to practice preventive medicine.

Infectious Diseases and Vaccinations

As we move from the past to the future, many infectious diseases have been reduced or eradicated. One of the most well-known has been smallpox, which now only exists in a few laboratories. Our hope was that infectious diseases would become a rare cause of morbidity and mortality, but with the reduction of many of these diseases have come a resurgence of others. The overuse of antibiotics and the emergence of antibiotic-resistant bacterial infections are of great concern, and HIV-AIDS , influenza and pneumonia remain significant causes of morbidity and mortality. On the positive side, new vaccinations have been developed that may protect the population from influenza and other serious illnesses.

Other Advances

Various types of minimally-invasive surgery techniques, some utilizing robots, allow doctors to operate with smaller incisions and more precision. 3-D printing is also finding more application in Medicine, e.g. in the creation of dental implants, prosthetics and more.

The Medical Home

There is increased focus on the concept of a patient-centered medical home. This primary care model is team-based, comprehensive and accessible.

Health Information Technology and Telemedicine

In the medical field, we are finally moving toward the increased use of health information technology. This has the potential to improve the quality of health care, increase safety and access to medical information, and even decrease costs. Health information technology includes the use of personal health records, in which patients themselves own and store their records (in various formats, such as paper or electronic files) and coordinate their health care. It also includes the use of electronic medical records, which are usually managed by healthcare providers in offices or institutions. This allows physicians to gain easy access to medical records when necessary and improve communication among healthcare providers. A challenge will be integrating the various electronic systems so that they communicate with each other. For example, it won't be helpful if a patient is transferred from one institution to another that cannot access records because the two systems don't "communicate" with each other. One of the additional concerns about electronic medical records is that of privacy. Yet another is cost in the short term. In the long term, however, it is believed that there will be significant monetary savings. In recent years Telemedicine has been playing a significant role in healthcare. It allows medical information and care to be delivered without geographic constraint.

The Physician Workforce

One noticeable trend in the medical field is the increased number of female physicians practicing medicine today. Some of them practice full time, while others practice part time. Nearly 50 percent of freshmen medical school classes are composed of women, whereas the numbers were far lower in the past. There is a projected shortage of physicians in the future. Increasing funding for medical and residency training programs, and utilizing all healthcare professionals efficiently and appropriately, are some ways to address the shortage.

Outsourcing

Outsourcing jobs has become a reality, and the medical field is no exception. Factors include the ability to access specialized care and technology as well as the shortage of physicians in certain fields, not to mention lower costs. It is no longer unusual for patients to have an X ray in one location only to have it read by a radiologist in another.

Prevention

I spoke to a representative in the Office of the Surgeon General, and she discussed its public health priorities, which are also listed on its website. There is an emphasis on prevention of disease, an approach that is close to my heart as a pediatrician. This involves promoting regular physical activity, healthy nutrition, and avoiding high-risk behaviors like smoking. She reminded me that it was also important for everyone to have regular checkups and preventive screenings, and to know their histories and personal risk factors. Another priority is emergency and other preparedness, which includes being prepared for pandemic infections as well as other emergency situations. Additional projects include eliminating health disparities and improving health literacy overall.

No one knows exactly what the nature of the medical profession will be in the future. The only thing we can know with certainty is that there will be constant discovery and change. If you enter into this field, you must be willing to embrace these facts and adapt to change. Our goals for the future should be that every individual will have access to good health care, and that we—as providers—will continue to seek knowledge and answers to improve the health of the community. We should strive to have better treatments for diseases such as cancer, heart disease, mental illnesses, autoimmune diseases, and AIDS. A medical career is filled with all kinds of hope and possibilities for the future. I hope that medicine will attract those with compassion, people who want to care for others, learn, ask the difficult questions, and search for solutions.

PART TWO

INTERVIEWS WITH SPECIALISTS

Although medical students, during the course of their training, rotate through a number of specialties, including internal medicine, pediatrics, family practice, surgery, psychiatry, neurology, and obstetrics and gynecology, they lack in-depth exposure to many others. It can be difficult for medical students to make decisions about their future careers without being aware of all the available options. As a medical student, I developed interest in a number of fields. During my orthopedics rotation, I imagined becoming an orthopedist. After "scrubbing up" and assisting with an appendectomy for the first time, I was certain I wanted to be a surgeon. During a rotation in forensic medicine, it seemed nothing else could be as exciting. And finally, after being exposed to pediatrics, I made up my mind that I wanted to care for children and adolescents.

I interviewed several physicians in various fields of medicine to illustrate the diversity of medical specialties and medical specialists. They pointed out the highlights and challenges of their fields and the medical profession in general. A few specialties are showcased more than once to present different experiences or points of view. I hope, as you read the in-depth interviews that follow, the many wonderful possibilities for your future in medicine will become more evident.

CHAPTER 10

INTERNAL MEDICINE

Internists (or internal medicine physicians) are doctors who specialize in the medical care of adults. Training to become an internist includes four years of medical school followed by a three-year residency program.

"You should go into medicine because you're going to help people and because it's a good profession," said Dr. Carol Salzman. "Don't choose this career to make millions of dollars."

Carol Salzman, an internist in private practice, told me that her father was a doctor, and she liked the fact that a medical career involved the combination of science and teaching. She initially considered a career in teaching and took several courses in education, but discovering later that she enjoyed the sciences more, she pursued a medical degree instead. She completed her medical training at Georgetown University and residency at George Washington, and now finds it rewarding to teach medical students rotating through her office, learning about the "practice of medicine."

I asked Dr. Salzman whether certain people are cut out to be internists, rather than surgeons or anesthesiologists, for example. "You certainly can do a better job if you tend to be a good listener, are willing to spend time with people, and don't need instant gratification," she said. "Most physicians choosing this field are probably inclined to have those skills. Certain aspects can be learned. The hardest part, I think, is learning how to take a good history from the patient and ask the right questions. If you don't listen to the patient, you may miss the diagnosis."

She then described her life as a physician. "Most of my patients are fifty years or older and come in for general care or acute problems. A smaller number have chronic medical problems. When dealing with very sick patients, it's hard not to take the worries home with you, but you learn how to deal with it over time." She told me that one of the most difficult, yet rewarding situations is helping a patient die comfortably while being with his or her family. "It's very hard," she said. "The art is finding what's best for each situation."

I asked her what else she found challenging about her field, and she said, "When you know a patient has something wrong but you can't figure out what it is and you don't know how to help them. In that case you keep trying, and sometimes you have to say, 'I'm stuck,' and refer them to someone else. It's important to learn what you know and not to feel threatened to say, 'I don't know,' when you don't." She recalled seeing a woman with a diffuse rash that resembled hives all over her body. There was no good explanation for the rash, and the patient had not had any known exposure to ticks. Dr. Salzman referred her to a dermatologist, who did a skin biopsy and drew blood tests for Lyme disease. The results were confusing because the blood tests were positive for Lyme disease and the biopsy was consistent with a lupus-type process. The patient was treated for Lyme disease, and the rash resolved. In this kind of situation, when the diagnosis is not clear-cut, the burden is usually placed on the internist (the primary care physician) to follow the patient and sort things out.

With respect to type of practice, there are many options available to internists. One can choose private practice, hospital-based medicine, academic medicine, or research. In fact, one of Dr. Salzman's colleagues joined the Peace Corps. Although there are many advantages to being in solo private practice, one of the downsides is having to take "call" more frequently, whereas one of the benefits of being in a group practice is being able to routinely share that call with others.

Dr. Salzman offered advice and insight to those pursuing medical careers. "I have learned how stressful it is to do this job and be a parent. If you are a parent or will become a parent soon, it's okay to realize that although it can be done, it is difficult and it's not simply a time-management issue. If you have a family, you've got to seriously think about the specialty you choose. Internal medicine might afford you some flexibility, whereas there may not be much flexibility if you choose surgery or obstetrics, for example. Medicine is a wonderful, prestigious career, but it also involves a lot of work and great commitment. I would not encourage anyone to go into medicine unless they were passionate about it. If you are, however, you should continue to pursue that path."

INTERNAL
MEDICINE

CHAPTER 11

OBSTETRICS AND GYNECOLOGY

An obstetrician-gynecologist is a physician who is a specialist in pregnancy, labor, and delivery, as well as the prevention and the treatment of diseases of the female reproductive system. Training includes four years of medical school followed by a four-year residency in obstetrics and gynecology.

"My dad was a family doctor," said Dr. Susan Hurson. "I used to go to the office and hospital with him and found it fascinating. He even took me into the emergency room." Dr. Hurson, an obstetrician-gynecologist in Washington, D.C., told me that both her parents were very supportive of her interest in medicine. She was an avid reader, volunteered at a local hospital as early as ninth grade, and had high hopes of pursuing a medical career.

"I graduated with a bachelor of science from Georgetown University," she said, "and because I didn't get into medical school right away, I spent several years working and doing research before reapplying to medical school. My first year was spent working at a New York City hospital following up on cancer patients, after which time I moved back to Washington, D.C., and became a receptionist for a large internal medicine group." Dr. Hurson told me that she found that particular job to be very stressful, although she learned a great deal. "Following that, I worked at the National Cancer Institute doing drug development, and because my job involved research and biostatistics, I found my science background to be very useful."

Eventually, she reapplied to medical school and was relieved to be accepted. "I found the first two years of medical school particularly interesting," she said. "There were challenges, of course, because of the high volume of material and because of my age. It was difficult being older than the other students and having to make new friends."

During medical school Dr. Hurson became interested in obstetrics and gynecology. "I considered different specialties," she said. "For example, I was interested in urology, but it was a male-dominated field, not very open to women. Obstetrics and gynecology, on the other hand, was also predominantly male, but the tide was changing. I also liked the residents and doctors. They were good teachers with good attitudes, so overall I enjoyed my rotation."

"The very first day I started my OB (obstetrics) rotation," she said, "the chief resident who was in charge said to me, 'Get your gloves on.' It was the first time I helped deliver a baby. I was so nervous, but I thought it was great." Dr. Hurson told me that later during her residency at a hospital in Washington, D.C., she encountered pregnant patients who had not had any prenatal care. "One patient in particular came to triage in active labor. We did an ultrasound, which revealed what we thought were twins with arms and legs entwined. We tried to figure out whether we should do a vaginal delivery versus a C-section and decided on vaginal. The first baby delivered, and I clamped the cord while I prepared for the second. The next baby came out, and I clamped the second cord and then waited for the placenta to detach. Something didn't look right. The placenta looked different and shiny. I suddenly realized it wasn't a placenta at all. It was a baby's bottom—a breech. Luckily, the baby was fine, but we were all stunned that there were three babies instead of two."

We later discussed the challenges physicians face. "A medical career is no longer always stable," she said. "Doctors change their work settings routinely—for example, from working in a hospital environment to private practice or to administration. There is less security in medical positions now, I think." She mentioned another downside, particularly in the field of obstetrics, namely the risk of malpractice suits and the high cost of malpractice insurance. However, on a positive note, Dr. Hurson told me that as long as one is willing to make compromises, physicians can create balance and enjoy the lifestyles they desire. She said there were many opportunities, such as working for a group practice, a hospital, or an HMO (health maintenance organization). She herself is a solo practitioner but cross-covers with a large group on weekends and holidays. She is happy with her decision to pursue a medical career. "In my heart of hearts," she said, "if I had not done medicine, it always would have bothered me. I would not have felt settled."

CHAPTER 12

GERIATRICS

A geriatrician is a physician who is a specialist in the care of the elderly. Training includes medical school, usually followed by a residency in internal medicine or family practice. Following residency, geriatricians usually have additional training in geriatric medicine and may complete a geriatric fellowship.

"Alzheimer's is a frustrating disease," said Dr. Maria Mannarino. "My patients were some of the most intelligent people with fruitful lives as scientists, politicians, and military officers, now slowly losing their capabilities and their memories." Dr. Mannarino worked at the National Institute on Aging at the National Institutes of Health (NIH) for many years, dividing her time between research and clinical medicine. She focused largely on patients with Alzheimer's disease. "Although it was challenging, I also found my work to be very rewarding," she said, "because I was able to spend significant time with the patients and their families, and offer them support when they needed it most."

I asked Dr. Mannarino what had inspired her to pursue a medical career. "My mother began studying medicine when she was nineteen years old," she said. "She then married and discontinued her studies, although she was always interested in holistic and alternative medicine. When I graduated from high school in Germany, my mother encouraged me to go into medicine. I became interested and even more so after meeting my mother's friend who practiced natural medicine. She allowed me to accompany her to study courses, and in my first year of medical school, she let me work in her practice. I learned how to deal with both geriatric and pediatric problems."

Dr. Mannarino graduated from a six-year medical program in Germany and then came to the United States for a pediatric residency at the Children's National Medical Center in Washington, D.C. "I enjoyed my residency very much," she said, "and I also met my husband, a neurosurgical resident, at Children's." Her husband took a position as a neurosurgeon at Duke University, and she herself was offered a fellowship there in pediatric neurosurgery. "After my fellowship, I had a daughter and took three years off to spend time with the family before returning to medicine to pursue research at the NIH. I began in general medicine and then switched to the National Institute on Aging where I studied geriatric problems, including Alzheimer's."

Dr. Mannarino sincerely hopes that more medical students will consider going into the field of geriatrics. "I really bonded with the patients and their families," she said. "I had one gentleman patient who spoke seven languages. He had lost most of his memory and could hardly communicate with his family. However, he had lived in Germany for some time, as I had, and we discovered we could speak to each other in German. We had lovely conversations." I asked whether the future was hopeful for patients with Alzheimer's disease. "I do see advances," said Dr. Mannarino. "At this time, there is nothing that can completely cure the disease, but we can do something to prolong a patient's well-being."

Dr. Mannarino has had a remarkable career, too. After twenty-five years at the NIH, she continued to utilize her experience in geriatrics and research, spending nine years as a consultant completing scientific reviews on breast and prostate cancer for the U.S. Army. She has enjoyed all aspects of her career and believes that she would have chosen the same path if she could start all over.

I then asked her about the challenges of balancing work and family life. "It was a struggle," she said. "I was required to travel a lot for work. I also had a husband and daughter, and when you have children at home, you have to be available. There wasn't much flexibility initially, but later on, we had flex time, so I could start work later and come home later when necessary."

Finally, I asked if she had any advice for students. "I think they should learn about the roadblocks, such as managed care and malpractice, now. Then, if they really want to be doctors and develop relationships with patients, they should absolutely do it."

We have heard from Dr. Mannarino, who completed her medical school training overseas and then continued her medical career in the United States. Next, let's learn what it's like to be a cardiologist.

CHAPTER 13

CARDIOLOGY

A cardiologist is a physician who specializes in the treatment of disorders of the heart and cardiovascular system. Training includes four years of medical school followed by a residency in internal medicine or pediatrics and then a fellowship in cardiology. I interviewed a cardiologist, an interventional cardiologist, and a pediatric cardiologist to give you a broader perspective of the practice of cardiology.

INTERVENTIONAL CARDIOLOGY

"It is a wonderful profession. I'm happy just knowing that I can play a part in making a difference in someone's life as a result of something I learned or something I know," said Dr. Ron Waksman, an interventional cardiologist. Today, Dr. Waksman travels all over the world to lecture and perform complicated cardiac procedures.

But did he always have aspirations of becoming a doctor? He told me that as a young boy in Israel, he used to dress up as a doctor for Purim (a Jewish holiday). Later, he became impressed by the medics in combat during the war. He wanted a profession that would incorporate science and technical skills, and still allow regular interaction with people. He made his decision to become a doctor while serving in the Israeli Army. After completing medical school and a residency (in internal medicine and cardiology) in Israel, he continued with a fellowship in interventional cardiology at Emory (in Atlanta) in the United States. He is now an associate director in the division of cardiology at the Washington Hospital Center in Washington, D.C.

The field of interventional cardiology is relatively new. In fact, the first coronary artery interventions were performed in the 1980s. According to Dr. Waksman, the goal of the field is to try to minimize unnecessary invasive surgeries when less-invasive procedures and surgeries can be done instead. In many cases, these procedures can significantly reduce the chances of dying after a heart attack if done early enough. Obviously, there have been great advances in the field. Still, more than a million people in the United States suffer from heart attacks each year and a significant number of people die from these attacks.

In the past, a patient with an acute myocardial infarction (heart attack) had few options. There was basically no treatment available other that rest and pain medication. In 1955, President Dwight Eisenhower suffered a heart attack in Denver, Colorado. At that time, patients were routinely kept in bed for up to six months, whereas now those without complications spend only a few days in the hospital. After his heart attack, President Eisenhower was treated with oxygen and medication, and was kept on bed rest for several weeks, after which time he was only allowed to sit up in a chair for a short while. After about seven weeks—sooner than most patients—he was allowed to begin walking again. Subsequent to his initial recovery, he required several hospitalizations and eventually died of heart failure in 1969 at the age of 78.

Treatment for this condition has changed dramatically. Recent advances have included the development of stents to keep arteries open, the first stents being used in humans in the 1990s. Today, a patient who has had a heart attack would probably be taken directly to the catheterization laboratory (or cath lab) for cardiac catheterization. A balloon angioplasty—a procedure that opens blocked arteries and restores blood flow to the heart—can be performed and a stent put in place. Fortunately, the success rate of the procedure is high.

Of course, I could write an entirely separate book on Dr. Waksman's testimonials alone. Leah Miller told me about the time that he saved her husband's life. A routine stress test done at his primary care doctor's office revealed some cause for concern. Mr. Miller was asked to set up an appointment for a cardiac catheterization procedure at his local hospital within the following few days. He called Dr. Waksman to discuss this with him, and Dr. Waksman recommended that he have the procedure done as soon as possible. In fact, he offered to perform the procedure himself at a hospital renowned for cardiac care. Indeed, cardiac catheterization demonstrated dangerous blockages of four arteries, requiring quadruple bypass surgery. After a discussion with Leah, arrangements were made immediately for a colleague who was a cardiac surgeon to perform the surgery, which was successfully completed just in time. Leah believes that if her husband had waited longer or had the procedure done at a different hospital, the outcome may have been very different.

Dr. Waksman believes that students and physicians considering a career in interventional cardiology should have good technical skills, good communication skills, and the passion to want to help people. "There are no shortcuts. One has to have a good all-around education and become proficient at general skills and knowledge. Students should also be curious, demonstrate creativity, and ask questions. They should not be hesitant to challenge their professors. Find a good mentor, and then once you have made the decision to enter this field, stay focused on it," he advised.

His career gives him great personal satisfaction because he feels that he can really make a difference by being able to intervene at critical times in a patient's life and potentially correct defects in an organ as vital as the heart. He described how the practice of medicine takes commitment and time and really defines one's life to some extent. "One has to understand that your life is not only your life." he said "It's also part of your patient's life. You also have to constantly ask yourself, 'Did I do the best that I could?'"

In the next section, you will read about a doctor who takes care of children with heart problems.

PEDIATRIC CARDIOLOGY

"I enjoy the complexity of the patients and the challenge that brings. It's never boring," said Dr. Frank Galioto, speaking of his life as a pediatric cardiologist. "Children are delightful, even the sick ones. Their families may be more difficult because of their anxiety, but you can't only treat the child; you have to work with the family as you make the diagnosis and plan treatment."

He spoke about the advances in the field. "It is constantly changing and evolving. We have greater ability to make prenatal diagnoses, and fetal echocardiography has opened a completely new arena so that more patients with serious cardiac defects survive now. The way we care for our patients today is very different from thirty years ago, so pediatric cardiologists have to maintain curiosity about their discipline and continually educate themselves."

Although Dr. Galioto's father was an anesthesiologist and he grew up in a medical home, he only made the decision to attend medical school in his junior year of college at Cornell. The decision to become a pediatric cardiologist was made while he was in medical school at New York Medical College, where he was inspired by two dynamic attendings who exposed him to the field. He remained in New York for his pediatric residency, working with a high volume of young patients, and then went to Baylor in Houston, Texas, where he completed a fellowship in pediatric cardiology. At Baylor, he had the opportunity to work with the well-known cardiac surgeon, Dr. Denton Cooley, to whom he frequently gave reports on patients. His primary teacher was Dr. Dan McNamara, a pioneer in pediatric cardiology and the chief of pediatric cardiology at Texas Children's Hospital. "Being there and working with that team made life even more exciting. We were cutting edge in therapy and diagnosis."

Dr. Galioto has spent more than thirty years in academic and private practice. He told me that he finds his work very rewarding. "I think we can make a positive difference with every patient encounter. In children with heart disease, we have effective treatments in almost all cases today. A patient who would have died fifty years ago now has a high likelihood of survival. Even if a child has an innocent murmur, I feel I am helping by giving the family the diagnosis and relieving them of their fears." He also said that he enjoys seeing patients whom he has known from birth and watching them grow and develop.

Next, I asked what he found challenging. "The most difficult part for me," he said, "is to tell a family that their child has a serious heart condition that will require a series of operations, and that they have a long road ahead of them." He explained that sometimes cardiologists seek another point of view or support from colleagues. "We routinely share all our difficult problems at a weekly conference so that our patients benefit from the opinions of the group as well." Dr. Galioto went on to explain that the challenges also made his work interesting. "Much of what we deal with in pediatric cardiology is unusual," he said, "because the diseases we see are not as common as those seen in adults. What's exciting about this field is that it's unpredictable. You have to be constantly alert, because the next patient may have something you have not seen before." He obviously loves his work but says it is often stressful and demanding. For many physicians, it can be difficult balancing their work and private lives. "You have to work at achieving the balance," said Dr. Galioto.

His advice to those considering a career in medicine is to find a field that will make you happy and that will best suit you. "Ease of learning comes when you enjoy what you study," he said. "Learn what you can about the innate challenges and rewards of the specialty you consider. This particular field is stressful in that you will be dealing with significant numbers of sick children." He believes that you must enjoy working with children, have empathy for other human beings, and should become adept at interacting with kids and families. "You should have an inquiring mind and be able to think in a systematic way. Don't go into medicine with the primary goal of making a huge salary. As in other medical specialties, it is no longer as financially rewarding as it was in the past, because of managed care," he said. "The physician's share of the healthcare dollar has decreased."

On the other hand, he derives great emotional satisfaction from working with children and believes he made the right career choice. "I don't know of any other specialty that would provide the same challenges. Also, although the children don't always acknowledge it, the families are generally quite appreciative of our efforts."

CARDIOLOGY AND PREVENTION

Heart disease is still the leading cause of death in the United States in spite of great advances made in the last few decades. In addition, symptoms in women are often not recognized until too late. Morbidity and mortality could be significantly reduced by sometimes simple lifestyle changes; unfortunately, this is not always easy to accomplish. Dr. Lisa Martin, a cardiologist and assistant professor of medicine at the George Washington University in Washington, D.C., is passionate about the issue. She believes that more attention should be placed on prevention, including the promotion of correct use of medication and a better lifestyle to achieve cardiac health. "I was very upset about seeing my patients having to go back for more and more procedures for coronary artery disease," she said. "I believe that we need to try to prevent the disease in the first place. A while ago, many articles were published on medications that reduced the risk of heart attacks, so at least we had something we could use for prevention."

She then added that another very important aspect of prevention, apart from medication, is a healthy lifestyle. Dr. Martin told me that she spends much of her time teaching her patients. "Patients have to understand their disease so that they can play significant roles in their treatment too," she said. "We're working on setting up a program where we would have ancillary people to deal with the nutritional and other aspects of heart disease and obesity."

Doctors can make a difference on an individual level with their patients, but they can also have a broader impact on community and public health. Heart disease, obesity, and other related problems are significant public health issues. "We've created programs where we have gone out into the communities and checked people's blood pressures and cholesterol levels, and helped with referrals when necessary," said Dr. Martin. "In that way, we can help promote health within the community."

She told me that she was also considering getting more involved in a government health policy program at George Washington University. "What we really need to do, though," she added, "is to go out into the schools and encourage physical education programs and start teaching children about healthy habits when they are still very young. To prevent coronary heart disease, it is best to begin early."

As an undergraduate student, Dr. Martin majored in applied mathematics at Harvard. In her year, there was only one other woman with the same major. "A few of my friends were considering medicine," she said, "so I took applied math related to biological sciences. I really enjoyed the section on cardiology and decided to pursue that specialty. Also, my uncle needed bypass surgery when he was only thirty-six years old, and that left an impression on me." After medical school, Dr. Martin completed an internal medicine residency at Johns Hopkins University School of Medicine and then a fellowship in cardiology at George Washington University School of Medicine. Today, she still believes she made the right decision when she chose this path.

Dr. Martin sees adults of all ages and once had the privilege of treating a patient who was 102 years old. "I see many of my patients over a long period of time," she said. "I enjoy playing this role in people's lives. Having patients come back feeling better and knowing that you're helping them is a wonderful thing. You have to consider that a gift."

We then discussed the issue of finding the balance between work and personal life. "Although it's a very busy life," said Dr. Martin, "one can find a balance." She told me that she has many interests outside of medicine, and she thoroughly enjoys ballet, modern dance, art, and building structures. "Some doctors work part time, which I did for a number of years. With more women in medicine today, I find there is more understanding and more flexibility. You have to work things out so that you find a balance." Dr. Martin and her husband worked things out by putting each other through medical school both financially and emotionally.

Dr. Martin has overcome many obstacles, and she has achieved significant accomplishments. Apart from her achievements within the medical field, she was a finalist for an astronaut position in 1984. "About a hundred applicants were chosen out of ten thousand," she said. "Some were pilots, and the rest were scientists applying for mission specialist." She also described herself as a goal-oriented person. "I have had a number of life-changing events, including surviving cancer; however, I have been able to adjust my life to keep on going. One has to be able to take what comes and go on with one's goals."

I asked if she had any advice for students considering a career in cardiology. "As my uncle, who was also a cardiologist, said, 'You've got to love it because you're going to spend so much time doing it.' Basically, you should enjoy working with people," Dr. Martin added, "and always remember that patients come first."

You have heard from three doctors who have given their different perspectives on the practice of cardiology. Next, let's hear from a neonatologist.

CHAPTER 14

NEONATOLOGY

A neonatologist is a physician who specializes in the care and treatment of newborns, particularly those who are premature or ill. After medical school, these doctors receive training in pediatrics followed by a fellowship in neonatology.

"When I was in New York, I debated between going into pediatric surgery or pediatrics," said Dr. Siva Subramanian, a neonatologist at Georgetown University Medical Center in Washington, D.C. "Because I was not completely sure, I decided to do a year of internship in general pediatrics, which I thought would give me a good knowledge base. In my second or third month, I was assigned to the NICU (neonatal intensive care unit). The very first night, I took care of a baby with ABO (blood type) incompatibility that needed an exchange transfusion. I was enthralled and was able to put the line in on the first shot. The exchange lasted two hours, and later, I saw the dramatic improvement in the baby. After that, it was neonatology all the way."

Dr. Subramanian completed his pediatric residency at the University of Maryland. "The chairman offered me the position of chief of the pediatric residency program," he said, "and was upset when I turned it down to pursue a neonatology fellowship instead." Dr. Subramanian is now professor of pediatrics and ob-gyn, and chief of the division of neonatology at the Georgetown University Medical Center.

Over the past two decades, he has witnessed significant improvements in technology, treatments, and outcomes in premature babies. I asked about the major advances in neonatology, and he said, "The biggest advance by far has been the use of surfactant in premature babies." Premature babies may lack surfactant, which is produced by the lungs, and this can lead to a serious breathing disorder known as respiratory distress syndrome. Treatment with surfactant in addition to oxygen and other measures can be lifesaving. "At Georgetown University Hospital, we were instrumental in conducting a multicenter study," said Dr. Subramanian. "There has been a reduction of almost 40 percent in mortality of premature babies with the use of surfactant. Another advance in the treatment of certain very ill babies with respiratory failure has been the use of inhaled nitric oxide in combination with high-frequency ventilation. The use of nitric oxide in these babies reduces their chances of needing ECMO (extracorporeal membrane oxygenation). Smaller, rapid ventilators, sensitive to the needs of tiny babies, are now available. Also, one of the recent advances is that of whole body cooling (hypothermia). Hypothermia has been shown to protect against brain injury, and when used within the first six hours in babies with hypoxic ischemic encephalopathy, it has been shown to decrease morbidity and mortality dramatically."

I asked about the challenges he faced in his career. "The greatest challenges for a neonatologist, I believe, are the ethical ones," he said. "For example, technology allows us to prolong life and perform complicated procedures in newborns and infants. We must make sure that we always consider the ethical implications and don't get trapped in the technology. The other challenges, such as the acute care and intricate procedures, I enjoy." Dr. Subramanian then told a story of two premature babies to illustrate the types of ethical dilemmas neonatologists face (see the section on ethics in Chapter 8).

I asked if he had any advice for medical students. For those students pursuing careers in obstetrics, pediatrics, or family practice, he strongly recommended a fourth-year medical school elective in the NICU at the hospital where they do their residencies. He told me that most of the medical students rotating through the neonatal intensive care unit are excited and scared, but within a week, they become more confident and develop a nice rhythm. They are directly supervised by residents at all times. And to all students interested in the field of neonatology, he said, "You have to like the intensity of care and feel comfortable having diffi-cult discussions with parents and dealing with issues of life and death."

CHAPTER 15

PEDIATRIC
INTENSIVE CARE

A pediatric intensivist (intensive care specialist, also known as critical care specialist) is a physician who specializes in the care of infants, children, and adolescents with critical or life-threatening illnesses and injuries. Training includes four years of medical school followed by residency and a fellowship.

"When I was a medical student, I did a rotation in the pediatric intensive care unit and found it to be very interesting," said Dr. Craig Futterman. "A pediatric cardiologist was running the unit because there were no intensive care specialists there at that time. In comparison, the technology wasn't as sophisticated as it is today, but the cardiologist showed me things I thought were fascinating. I saw how one could literally save lives, and I decided that's what I wanted to do."

Dr. Futterman, a pediatric intensivist in Northern Virginia, knew that he wanted to become a doctor since he was six years old. "My own pediatrician was the one who inspired me," he said. "My dad was a disc jockey, and when I was very young, he did a recording interviewing my siblings and me. On the recording I said that I wanted to be a pediatrician."

Dr. Futterman then said that although he enjoyed his pediatric residency and the outpatient clinic, he knew that if he did that for the rest of his life, he would become bored. He decided instead to pursue a career in pediatric intensive care, so after his pediatric residency, he went on to complete an anesthesia residency followed by a pediatric critical care fellowship.

I asked Dr. Futterman about some of the challenges he has faced. "One of the most difficult cases for me," he said, "was the case of a baby in our intensive care unit who was born with anencephaly (absence of a large part of the brain). The situation was so unusual that the case was made public after it went to court. The baby's mother wanted everything done to keep her baby alive no matter what. Our team, on the other hand, felt that at some point it became futile and was not fair to the baby or anyone else. We decided to pursue legal action, but we lost the case in court. We continued with treatment, and the baby lived for about two years. That situation was very difficult and sad for my nursing staff, my colleagues, and me."

However, many more of his experiences are rewarding and make the hard work and long hours worthwhile. Dr. Futterman told me about one of those experiences. "A young child had a serious heart defect requiring an operation," he said. "Immediately after surgery, he kept arresting and was in our hospital intensive care unit for several months. He was a scrawny baby, and we didn't think he could survive much longer. Ten years later, at a reunion picnic for cardiac patients and their doctors, a tall boy jumped into the surgeon's arms and gave him a big hug. We had never forgotten our patient and all the nights we spent struggling to keep him alive. On that particular day, the look of gratitude in his parents' eyes was one that convinced me all the hours spent in the hospital were worth it."

Dr. Futterman told me that he likes the challenge and the satisfaction of treating heart surgery as well as other very sick patients. "As an intensivist, you have to be able to tolerate uncertainty and risk to a greater extent than in many other specialties," he said. "You must also be able to work as a team with other doctors and nurses. Our nurses are incredible people who are on the front line and do a great job." He told me that the most difficult part of his job is not having enough time with his family. "What I hadn't taken into consideration was the busy lifestyle. If you are interested in a career in intensive care, you must be aware that you will work long hours and frequently be up all night."

We then discussed some of the advances in his field. "I think one of the biggest breakthroughs has been related to vaccination," he said. "The hemophilus influenza vaccine, for example, has markedly reduced the number of patients with diseases like meningitis and has practically eliminated epiglottitis. Other advances have come from improvement in technology. The intensive care unit is a high-tech environment. Our ability to oxygenate and ventilate patients has improved. Computer-controlled ventilators, newer monitoring devices, and bedside testing have all made taking care of patients easier. A handheld device now allows doctors to have blood, gas, and electrolyte results within about three minutes instead of an hour or more."

We discussed how medical care was evolving and what the future would hold. The field of pharmacogenetics is fascinating and has significant implications with respect to the treatment of patients. Dr. Futterman said that work is being done to study how different people respond to medications based on their individual genetic makeup. "For example," he said, "a certain percentage of people lack the enzyme to break codeine down to morphine. Having this knowledge will allow us to target medications to a patient's genetic profile. Scientists are also looking at how patients respond to sepsis and injury." He said that another advance in the future will be the increased use of wireless monitoring. "It will become more common and more dependable, simplifying patient monitoring. Also, computerized data gathering will be instrumental in allowing us to look back on data and find patterns that may help us improve care."

"One of the biggest priorities at our hospital," said Dr. Futterman, "is the 'safety push.' We literally have physicians and other healthcare providers go over a checklist before starting any procedure, including placing intravenous lines and drawing blood. This is similar to what airline pilots do before taking off on a flight. At the hospital, we call it a procedure pause. This has significantly reduced errors and cost." Dr. Futterman told me that although some physicians have had trouble with this (possibly because of ego), the annual number of procedural errors has decreased dramatically. "The procedure pause has saved lives," he said, "and that's what it is all about. Our work with central lines has changed. The physician's insertion technique and the way nurses enter the line to draw blood and give medications have dramatically reduced bloodstream infections. This has saved lives and reduced costs."

I could tell that Dr. Futterman was passionate about his field and wondered if he would advise others to pursue a medical career. "I would definitely advise students to pursue medicine if that's what interests them," he said. "The biggest problem I anticipate, however, is that the enormous cost of medical school will keep some good people out of the field."

In parting, as we reflected on how much progress has been made and what we hoped for the future, he added that he wished for universal health care and access to good medical care for all children. "When one sees a four-year-old having surgery for a congenital heart condition that was never diagnosed because the child hadn't seen a doctor," he said, "it is terribly sad."

Dr. Futterman described his experiences and gave us insight into the life of a pediatric intensivist. In the next chapter, you will hear about the very different experiences of a geneticist.

CHAPTER 16

GENETICS

A geneticist is a physician or scientist who is a specialist in the field of genetics (i.e., the diagnosis and treatment of hereditary and genetic disorders). Training typically includes four years of medical school, followed by a residency and then a fellowship.

Dr. Kenneth Rosenbaum, an ex-baseball player, made a comparison between the game and clinical genetics. "As a relief pitcher, one has to have a certain mentality," he said. "We could be called upon at a moment's notice, and we had to be ready quickly."

Dr. Rosenbaum, a geneticist, is director of the Center for Prenatal Evaluation in the Division of Genetics and Metabolism at Children's National Medical Center and an associate professor of pediatrics at the George Washington University Medical Center in Washington, D.C. He enrolled in a seven-year combined college/medical school program at the University of Louisville, Kentucky, and learned quickly that the study of genetics and malformations interested him more than general pediatrics. He enjoyed the challenge and unpredictability, and found that he had an ability to remember facts and make diagnoses quickly. "I was the kind of person who could memorize citations easily," he said. By the time Dr. Rosenbaum finished medical school, he had completed a three-year student fellowship. After medical school, he did a three-year pediatric residency and then a fellowship in genetics.

I wondered whether anyone had inspired him to choose a medical career. "I had an uncle who was an orthopedic surgeon and also went to Louisville, but I was somewhat self-motivated," he said. "In medical school, I received a phone call from someone at the hospital, asking me to see a baby with a malformation. I took a look at the baby and told the group that he had a 'clover-leaf' skull. I remember how surprised they were that a medical student could know that. That's when I knew genetics was my calling."

Dr. Rosenbaum has become accustomed to being called at a moment's notice, too. "The best part of my job is going to the hospital and diagnosing and treating patients with malformations," he said. "It is important for the parents to have access to someone with experience. Geneticists are a resource for the families as well as for the pediatricians." He told me that the most challenging part of his job is being on call and working as hard as he did twenty or thirty years ago when he was much younger. "Although many students are interested in genetics, today they more often pursue research rather than clinical genetics," he said, "so my daily routine is no longer typical of physicians in this specialty." Dr. Rosenbaum divides his time between seeing patients in outpatient clinics, doing hospital visits, and emergency newborn consults. The majority of his patients have birth defects, neurofibromatosis, or Down syndrome.

We spoke about genetic disorders and the significant breakthroughs in the field. "A genetic disorder is one that is determined by alterations in the genome, which may interact with environmental components and other genes," he said. He went on to explain that although 100 percent of cancer is genetic, only about 15 percent is inherited, while the other 85 percent is caused by "insults" to genes that occur after birth.

Dr. Rosenbaum also adamantly believes that genetics is an essential component of every medical specialty. "Technology has revolutionized the field of genetics and our ability to make diagnoses," he said. New advances include the regular use of microarrays that allow scientists to identify particular gene sequences and analyze a larger numbers of genes more quickly, which significantly helps in the diagnosis of genetic disorders that we were unable to diagnose in the past.

The human genome project, which involved the sequencing of every gene in humans, has brought with it great hope as well as ethical concerns. We have reached an era of commercialization of genetic information. People can now pay to receive their personal genetic "maps" (genome). Should patients have access to their genomes, and could this knowledge help or hurt them? What about the privacy issue, and who should be allowed to have this information? Would knowledge about your risk for developing a certain disease later in life affect health insurance coverage or employment opportunities? We have yet to see how people will avail themselves of this technology in the future.

If you are considering the field of genetics, Dr. Rosenbaum advises some caution. He says that the lifestyle of a clinical geneticist is extremely busy. "I've spent much of my life not being available outside of work," he said.

He went on to say that the routine of a physician in research was very different, and there may be more opportunity to balance work, family, and extracurricular life. I then asked him what character traits suited someone in his field. "They are the same that would suit a pediatrician," he said. "Pediatricians and geneticists are usually accessible. They are warm people who relate to families and children well. They should have good memory skills and enjoy detective work. He compared making a diagnosis to solving a puzzle, working backwards from the answer. You see the patient with the malformation, and then you have to work back towards the genetic root of the problem. Although Dr. Rosenbaum had some hesitation when asked if he would advise anyone to pursue this field, he was quite clear when he said, "For me, it's been a thrilling time."

CHAPTER 17

RADIOLOGY

A radiologist is a physician who is a specialist in the interpretation of radiological images for the prevention and treatment of disease and disorders. Training typically involves four years of medical school followed by a radiology residency. Radiologists may then choose to sub-specialize by pursuing a fellowship in one of various fields, such as neuroradiology or interventional radiology.

"Medicine is a wonderful career, which promotes independence and offers a broad range of opportunities and tremendous job satisfaction," said Dr. Bernard Gero, a radiologist in California. His inspiration to pursue a medical career came from his own general practitioner. "When I was a child, our family doctor would come over for house calls," he continued, "and it was obvious to me that he was someone our family could lean on."

When in medical school, Dr. Gero would go down to the X ray department with frequency. "I found radiology to be fascinating," he said, "and interventional radiology in particular piqued my interest. The work was intricate, involving catheters and needles. It was a field that was both practical and cerebral." After medical school, Dr. Gero completed a four-year radiology residency at St. Luke's Roosevelt in New York and then a two-year fellowship in neuroradiology at Yale.

"The most exciting part for me is working through a clinical problem together with the patient's physician to come to a clear diagnosis," said

Dr. Gero. "Discussing the imaging and which studies to do—and then interpreting those tests in conjunction with the clinical picture—can help the treating doctor develop the best course of action for the patient." Then, he told me that a diagnosis he has frequently made is that of a subdural hematoma. "A patient may be skiing, for example," said Dr. Gero, "when he falls and bumps his head. His symptoms may be mild and then improve temporarily. A week or more later, he has a headache or may not feel well. We do a head CT scan and find a hematoma."

I asked Dr. Gero about the biggest challenges that he faces in this field. "It is the constant change that is occurring," he said, "but that's also what makes it so interesting. I have to keep up to date with the explosion of new information and technology, and it keeps me challenged. As the computer age has evolved, medicine has embraced it, and I have found it to be wonderful and more efficient."

Next, we discussed some of the significant advances in the field of radiology. With the advent of PACS (picture archiving and communications systems), radiologists are moving away from film to computer (digital) imaging, which could potentially speed up and improve the accuracy of readings. The ability to perform positron-emission tomography (PET) and a CT scan simultaneously enables functional and anatomic imaging to be combined. This method has only recently become available for the clinical evaluations of patients with cancer, dementia, and heart problems. Another advance in technology has been in the form of CT coronary angiography, which utilizes scanners that take faster pictures and therefore have the ability to take CT images of the coronary arteries. Teleradiology has become a growing area in which radiological images such as X rays and CT scans can be read from a distance.

I asked Dr. Gero whether he would advise students to enter the medical profession, and he answered, "I would still advise them to do so, with some caveats. The first is to be aware of the financial implications. A medical education is long and costly and the debt can become burdensome to young physicians wanting to start a career and possibly get married and have children. It is also important for students to set their sights appropriately and go into medicine for the right reasons and to keep pace with the constant changes in the field." He stressed that we all have to come to terms with the fact that medicine is different from what it was a few decades ago, and we have to focus on the present rather than dwell on the past. "A medical profession is a noble profession that offers tremendous diversity, including clinical or pharmaceutical research, biotechnology, managed care, or policy. The field is vast and there are many opportunities for physicians other than primary care medicine."

"One of the things I enjoy about the field of radiology is the communication with other physicians," he said. "I interact with almost every other specialty, including obstetricians needing ultrasounds, ENT specialists evaluating for sinusitis, psychiatrists concerned about Alzheimer's, and pediatricians ordering chest X rays. I know most of the physicians in the community because they all refer patients to radiology at some point. I find it very stimulating because it keeps me interested in a broad range of medicine."

Dr. Gero has now given us a look into the field of radiology. Next, let's hear from a plastic surgeon.

CHAPTER 18

PLASTIC SURGERY

A plastic surgeon is a surgeon who specializes in the treatment of disfigurement or scarring of the face or body, as well as certain skin lesions, and is also qualified to perform cosmetic and reconstructive surgery.

"My goal is not only to have a good result technically, but also to have a patient who is happy," said Dr. Armin Karl Moshyedi, a plastic surgeon in Bethesda, Maryland. He told me that his father was a physician, as were his two older brothers. However, it was during his clinical rotation in surgery at the University of Maryland medical school that he found his comfort zone. "Surgery fit my personality," he said, "and halfway through my general surgery residency, I made the decision to specialize in plastic surgery. During my residency, I had a lot of experience with breast cancer, and as a fellow, I took care of breast surgery patients from a reconstructive standpoint. As a plastic surgeon one of my responsibilities was to guide patients with respect to their best options after mastectomy."

Dr. Moshyedi told me that he had a wonderful mentor, Dr. Luis Vasconez, who taught him much about the humanitarian side of medicine. "We're lucky to have our patients come to us and put their trust in us, particularly for elective procedures," he said. "They in turn deserve good customer service." He told me that plastic surgeons should be customer-service-oriented and humble. They should also be able to put themselves in patients' shoes and understand things from their point of view. He believes that many of these skills may not come naturally to surgeons but may be learned. It should go without saying that they must be technically oriented as well. "People see exactly what you did and will judge you thereby. You have to accept that they may complain about things that are out of your control. It therefore helps if they have realistic expectations. Don't try to overstate what you can do."

Dr. Moshyedi believes that some physicians are attracted to the glamour of the field, but those physicians are usually "weeded out" early in their careers. "A plastic surgeon needs to be a team player," he said. "For example, combined reconstructive procedures are done together with a general surgeon or orthopedist, and the plastic surgeon may have to adjust his or her schedule and wait for the surgeon—sometimes for a long time. Ideally, the plastic surgeon should be affable, patient, and available. In non-ideal situations, power struggles may occur between the plastic surgeon and the general surgeon."

He then started to describe the biggest challenges that he faces in this field. "If a patient has a complication," he said, "I also have to live with it. I will then follow up with the patient frequently—sometimes every other day—for medical reasons and to reassure them. The goal is to have a healthy and happy patient. Another challenge is the preoperative evaluation or discussion. It is not going to change what I do technically, but it will affect their understanding; and if patients are more knowledgeable about the procedures and outcomes. they tend to do better. When I was practicing general surgery, I wasn't as aware of the customer service aspect of medicine. As a plastic surgeon, I learned a whole new set of doctor skills."

Dr. Moshyedi spoke about the significant advances in the field, including the improvements in microvascular surgery techniques, using free flaps for saving limbs among these improved techniques. According to Dr. Moshyedi, it's an exciting field in which you can specialize and tailor your practice to suit your skills and your lifestyle.

Here, Dr. Moshyedi described some of his experiences as a plastic surgeon. In the next chapter, Dr. Jach will take us into the world of the anesthesiologist.

CHAPTER 19

ANESTHESIOLOGY

Anesthesiologists are physicians who specialize in airway management, pain management, and the care of the surgical patient. They possess a high degree of technical skill, which allows them to perform intubations as well as other complicated procedures.

"You have to be able to be calm under stress," said Dr. Michael Jach. "Ninety percent of what I do is routine and 10 percent is very exciting. Usually, the most exciting times happen when you least expect it. Malignant hyperthermia, for example—when it happens, all hell breaks loose, and if you don't know what to do, you could have a dead patient on your hands."

Dr. Jach is an anesthesiologist at a local hospital in Maryland. After completing medical school in South Africa, he sat for his ECFMG and VQE (visa qualifying exam) in South Africa. He then moved to the United States where he passed the FLEX exam before practicing medicine here. "My dad was a doctor. All I ever wanted to be was a doctor. I knew it from a very young age—as far back as I can remember. I had no second choice."

He described the following clinical situation, one which only solidified the fact that although anesthesiologists put patients to sleep, they themselves need to remain extremely alert. "A patient comes in with a ruptured abdominal aneurysm. He is brought to the operating room, and his bleeding is initially controlled. All of a sudden, the rupture extends;

blood is rising and spilling over the side of the bed! The situation is that of controlled chaos. The nurses are calling the blood bank for O-negative blood (the universal donor). There is a rush to get more help. At least two or three anesthesiologists are trying to get access to veins. After trying all we can and seeing no positive response, we find ourselves faced with an ethical dilemma—at what point do we stop resuscitating?"

I quickly learned that this is one of the most difficult clinical decisions these doctors must make. I wondered how other doctors dealt with this stress and how they were able to calm themselves so that they could concentrate on their next patients. "Whatever happens," said Dr. Jach, "even if there's a bad outcome, you've got to be able to accept it and put it behind you." He then compared the experience to being a pilot flying a plane. "Just as every flight has to be treated with the same thoroughness, so does every patient need to receive your full attention and the identical high standard of care."

Continuing our conversation, I asked him what challenged him most. "I find open heart surgery very challenging, but I enjoy it. In a way, you are putting someone in a controlled death situation on a bypass machine. The beginning of the case is most stressful because usually the patient is compromised and you don't know how they will respond to the anesthesia. The other difficult time can be getting them off bypass, especially in the case of elderly or frail patients who may need more drug support. I definitely have more adrenaline going during those times."

He told me that because this is a stressful field and because doctors may have such a full caseload, they sometimes forget that the patient is a human being. Curious, I asked Dr. Jach how he himself avoided falling into that trap. "I always imagine me being in the patient's position. These are the most anxious patients. The idea of being on a bypass machine is frightening, so I try to allay their anxiety. I love dealing with patients—the human nature and emotional side. I also have to deal with the patient's family and explain to them that their loved one is going to have intravenous lines (IVs), catheters, and chest tubes coming out of their body, but after a few days, they may be well enough to go home."

Some anesthesiologists, like Dr. Jach, work in hospital settings; others work in freestanding clinics, completing minor, low-risk procedures such as endoscopies or light-sedation surgeries. Dr. Jach finds that less stimulating, but he does find balance by spending time treating patients with chronic pain. "I try to tailor my treatment to what is acceptable to the patient. By incorporating alternative therapies such as yoga and acupuncture, I try to minimize the use of conventional narcotics and invasive procedures, which could have serious side effects. Surgery is a last resort."

Finally, Dr. Jach gave advice for students considering this field. "You have to enjoy being part of a team as opposed to being a solo practitioner. You will be working with surgeons, residents, nurses, techs. You are basically providing a service to the surgeon and the patient, so don't think that you are going to stand out like a superstar. The key to liking your job is to find balance. You can find balance within your career, for example, by working in 'open heart' as well as pain management, and you can find balance by having interests outside of medicine, too. Anesthesiology is a profession that is well-reimbursed, but high-risk. If things go wrong, they can go terribly wrong—we're talking severe neurological damage or death. The good news is that the drugs and monitoring have improved so that the risks have decreased. It's an excellent profession, but you have to be ready to accept that you can do everything by the book and still have a negative outcome." Closing, I asked if there were any final words of advice for students, and he responded, "Do what you love doing. Ultimately, that will be the most rewarding."

CHAPTER 20

DERMATOLOGY

A dermatologist is a physician who specializes in diseases and disorders of the skin and related structures. Training includes four years of medical school followed by a residency.

"To be a good dermatologist, one has to be a detective," said Dr. Laurence Miller, a dermatologist in private practice in Maryland. "In medical school, the dermatology professor used to present patients to us in an amphitheater. The professor would bring in a patient, then call a student down, and read the patient's history; for example, 'This is a thirty-two-year-old construction worker who developed a terrible rash on both feet. His fungal studies were negative. Would you like to ask him any questions?' The student, Robert, asked the patient what part of construction he was involved in and found out that he worked with cement. Robert diagnosed dermatitis (skin rash) and upon asking further questions, found out that the man had no personal or family history of eczema. He did, however, work in his boots all day while cement was being poured. It turned out that his feet became wet as the cement soaked through his boots. He had developed an allergic contact dermatitis from the cement. Further testing revealed that he was sensitive to chromium (chromate), a component of cement."

"We saw many patients with the professor, and the students enjoyed solving the various cases. They were like Sherlock Holmes mysteries," said Dr. Miller. "That's when I became interested in dermatology."

Recalling another more recent clinical situation, Dr. Miller began, "A man came into my practice on a cold, gray day in January. He had his right arm in a sling and a rash on his palm. The man had no idea how he had contracted the rash. He hadn't done any work on the house and had no particular hobbies. He had not been exposed to chemicals and had no history of eczema. I found this perplexing. The patient told me that I was no better than the orthopedist at making a diagnosis." The orthopedist had diagnosed tennis elbow, although the man had never played tennis. However, he did have severe pain in his elbow, so he walked around with his arm in a sling. All of a sudden, Dr. Miller recalled something he had seen in an old Jerry Lewis movie and asked the patient, "Did someone send you a case of oranges, and did you by any chance use a handheld juice maker to squeeze them?" he asked. To the patient's amazement, Dr. Miller was right; the patient had indeed spent a weekend squeezing a large number of oranges. He had developed tennis elbow from the repetitive motion and dermatitis from the friction of the orange rind on the palm of his hand. Another mystery solved!

"Although dermatology is a visual specialty, taking a good history is extremely important," said Dr. Miller. "You really need to spend adequate time with a patient to make a proper diagnosis." Dr. Miller primarily practices medical dermatology, but he also does some cosmetic procedures. "The bottom line is making people happy," he said. "From time to time teenage patients come in with severe acne. On the first visit, I find they won't make eye contact with me. As their acne gets better, they appear happier, and they start walking taller and looking me in the eye. It's very rewarding. There was another situation in which a male psychiatrist came to me for a consultation. He had a deep groove between his eyebrows and his patients had complained that he looked angry. With cosmetic treatment the groove disappeared and his facial expression softened. He also felt happier and found that he could treat his patients more effectively."

Dr. Miller told me that dermatologists are frequently required to practice "psychotherapy." He is acutely aware of how dermatological conditions can affect patients in all ways. For example, teenagers with psoriasis may avoid social situations because of shame. "In some situations, like psoriasis, there is no cure, but there is no patient to whom I've said, 'I can't help you,'" said Dr. Miller. One time, he was asked for advice from a patient whose girlfriend had herpes; the man was having second thoughts about marrying her. After a long discussion in the office, he weighed the benefits of being with the right person against the risks that could be minimized and elected to marry her. The patient was so grateful that he thanked Dr. Miller with a bottle of champagne.

Always curious, I asked Dr. Miller what lessons he had learned during his years in practice. "I had two professional shocks," he said. "I was under the impression that with great diligence, study, and research, I could cure everybody, and I've found out that's not the case. My second realization is that in spite of being compassionate and caring, not everyone will like me. On the other hand, I have been practicing for thirty-six years, and I still enjoy it. Some doctors make a lot of money seeing large numbers of patients. I'm not burned out, because I take my time."

Dr. Miller advises any student interested in dermatology to do an elective rotation in a doctor's office. "Following the doctor from room to room and observing the one-on-one doctor-patient relationship—like a fly on the wall—is invaluable and may ultimately shape the way you practice medicine."

CHAPTER 21

MEDICINE IN THE MILITARY

To get a glimpse into medicine in the military, I interviewed Colonel Phillips, a military physician who studied osteopathic medicine. Starting our conversation, he discussed the unique path he took to a medical career.

"I knew from the time I was in third grade that I wanted to be a doctor," said Colonel Stephen Phillips. "I went to a high school with a college prep curriculum, and my guidance counselor was very supportive. I also attended a premed day at Ohio State, where I learned about osteopathic medicine, and I became interested. There were no doctors in my family. My dad was a pilot in the U.S. Air Force, so we moved frequently—until third grade when we remained in Columbus, Ohio, for some time. I applied to Ohio State for college because they offered me the best scholarship, and I was happy that I was accepted."

Then, I asked Dr. Phillips about his major in college. "I majored in chemistry because I was advised to do so at the premed day. They indicated that this would increase my chance of getting into medical school." Only later did he find out that advice may not have been completely accurate. "As a college freshman, I was living in dorms. It was a big change from being the third of nine kids attending an all-boy Catholic high school. During that first year, I didn't let my studies interfere with my [overall] education, so I learned a lot about life. As a result, my grades were poor. I thought to myself, 'If I didn't become a doctor, I would possibly become a priest.' Those plans changed quickly when I met my girlfriend, who is now my wife. One of my chemistry teaching assistants said to me, 'You had better think of another profession because you're never going to be a doctor with grades like this.' I started thinking and realized he was right. I had to knuckle down and do better. In my sophomore year, I was taking organic and physical chemistry, and it hit me again that I was not going to go to medical school with those grades. I imagined that if I didn't get into medical school, I'd have to become a chemist, and I didn't like chemistry." Dr. Phillips then revealed an incident that occurred in his freshman year and affected him significantly. "There was a girl who was pregnant and suicidal, and a friend and I stayed up all night counseling her. I found out that there is a lot more to life than what I was doing. I realized that I wanted to be in a people-helping profession."

Dr. Phillips and his wife both joined a service organization, and the advisor happened to be the head of the department of social work. "I told him I wanted to change my major to social work. He said, 'You've talked to me. I know you've wanted to be a doctor since you were a little kid. If you enjoy working with people, change your major to something you're interested in, and if you don't get into medical school, come and see me then.' In the fall of my sophomore year, I changed my major to a double major in sociology and psychology. Since I was still pursuing a medical career, I also had to do chemistry and physics." Dr. Phillips told me that right after he switched his major and changed his attitude, he studied harder, his grades improved, and he soon achieved straight As. He later graduated with a double major in sociology and psychology and a minor in zoology.

"I had looked into osteopathic medicine," he told me. "Here, the philosophical approach emphasizes the whole person. It also incorporates manipulative medicine and the therapeutic nature of touch. Importance is placed on primary care and being a well-rounded physician. My number one choice for medical school was Ohio University College of Osteopathic Medicine, and I was accepted. To pay for school, I applied to the Health Professions Scholarship Program."

Notably, Dr. Phillips completed his residency at the Eisenhower Army Medical Center in Georgia. "My first assignment was at Fort Riley, Kansas, where I was to be a full-service family practice physician. Not long after that, Saddam Hussein invaded Kuwait, and I was pulled to become a surgeon for an armor battalion." Dr. Phillips explained that all physicians in the military, including internists, family physicians, and pediatricians, are referred to as surgeons. "In January 1991, we were deployed to Saudi Arabia for Operation Desert Shield and Operation Desert Storm," he said. "There I was, the primary care physician for about five hundred men, working out of the back of an armored vehicle."

Recalling one particular situation during his service, Dr. Phillips stated, "We had a tank driver who lifted his head out of the tank. When the turret (rotating part of the tank) turned, it hit his head, and he was severely injured. I stabilized his cervical spine, made sure he had an airway, and treated him with pain medication. We then called a helicopter to take him to the combat support hospital." He told me the advanced trauma support training he had undergone was helpful and that all military physicians complete a combat casualty care course at the beginning of residency.

Colonel Phillips is currently assistant chief of the Medical Corp Branch at Army Human Resources Command and is stationed in Virginia. He matches physicians to army positions in terms of type of practice and location. He told me that his next position will involve commanding a combat support hospital based out of Kentucky.

In closing, I asked the Colonel if he had any advice for students. "An advisor once told me that it must be really awful to be so focused on what you're going to do in the future, you're not having fun with what you're doing today. The journey's important. I adjusted my attitude and realized that it was kind of interesting to learn about chemistry, not just because I had to get an A for medical school. So if you're thinking that the process of going through medical school takes long, make the decision that you're going to enjoy actually being a medical student."

Colonel Phillips has shared his interesting experiences and given insight into the life of a physician in the military. For more information on the Health Professions Scholarship Program, see Chapter 6.

CHAPTER 22

ALLERGY/IMMUNOLOGY

An allergist/immunologist is a physician who specializes in the diagnosis and treatment of allergy and disorders of the immune system. Allergies indicate sensitivity of the immune system to a "foreign" protein, which means the two aspects—allergy and immunology—are related. Training includes four years of medical school followed by a residency in internal medicine or pediatrics and a fellowship in allergy and immunology.

"Medicine is a great profession," said Dr. Shelby Josephs. "I used to tell my wife how lucky I was because all my life I never minded coming to work." Dr. Josephs, an allergist in private practice in Maryland, told me that he always wanted to be a doctor. Like so many others I interviewed, his father was a physician, a pediatrician in this case. Shelby noticed that his father worked hard without complaining and really seemed to enjoy what he was doing. He nicknamed his father's colleagues, all of whom he liked, the bow-tie and brown-shoes types. Obviously, growing up in the presence of his father and his friends had a significant influence on his career choice.

During his medical school training at Duke University, he became interested in allergy and immunology, and found the head of the program, Dr. Rebecca Buckley, to be an excellent mentor who ran a strong program. Dr. Josephs next went to St. Louis Children's Hospital to complete a residency in pediatrics, and then returned to Duke for his fellowship in allergy and immunology. "I was attracted to immunology because it was a budding field in the early 1970s," said Dr. Josephs. "In addition, I was exposed to good role models at Duke University. They had excellent teachers and clinicians and performed world-famous research."

Having recently interviewed two surgeons and an anesthesiologist, I imagined the routine and lifestyle of an allergist to be very different. I asked Dr. Josephs what character traits he thought were necessary for someone interested in the field of allergy and immunology. "Ideally, they should be interested not only in the day-to-day manifestations of allergy," he said, "but also in the basic science, which can help us improve our therapies and guide us in making decisions about treatment options. Allergists must have curiosity. Much of what we do is detective-type work. One of the challenges is that we see a lot of the same things over and over, so we have to stay alert in order to recognize the unusual." He told me about a patient he saw who had eaten a fish meal and developed unusual headaches and paresthesia. She had a negative medical workup at a hospital, but she was believed to have some allergies, so she was referred to Dr. Josephs. After a detailed evaluation, he diagnosed her as having ciguatera toxicity, a fish-borne poisoning. As was expected, the patient got better with time.

Although he has enjoyed his career and believes he made the correct choice at the time, Dr. Josephs did discuss some of the reservations he had about a medical career in general. "Many years ago, if my kids told me they wanted to become doctors, I would have been very happy," he said. "Today, I would have some reservation and anxiety. There are many more external impositions placed on doctors and practices now, including higher costs, a larger amount of paperwork, and more regulations. I think the concept of solo practice will be rare in the future, and most doctors in private practice will work for big groups or the government. It is also difficult and time-consuming dealing with insurance companies, some of which don't seem to have any stake in either the doctor's or the patient's satisfaction. An additional concern is the debt that doctors incur during training. Four years of medical school followed by a three-year residency and then a three-year fellowship amounts to ten years of training, the first half of which one makes little or no salary." Both of us agreed, however, that the rewards of practicing medicine are far more than monetary, and although it is important that you are aware of the sacrifices you need to make, the ability to help and affect people in so many positive ways makes a medical profession well worth it.

"Unlike surgery, allergy is a field in which you can have regular hours and plan your lifestyle more easily," he said. "Although you can position yourself to spend more time in the hospital—to deal with drug allergies, for example—most allergists don't spend much time in the hospital and have few night calls. As an allergist, one can definitely find a balance between work, family, and extracurricular activities."

Later, Dr. Josephs spoke about some of the advances in the field of allergy and immunology. "There have been great advances," he said, "in terms of basic science application to allergy and the understanding of the physiology. The use of inhaled steroids has made a big difference in the treatment of patients with allergies. Primary care doctors are prescribing these medicines to patients with allergies, and many times, I'll only see the patients who don't respond, and they probably don't have allergy. Many of those patients end up having chronic sinusitis, nonallergic rhinitis, gastroesophageal reflux disease, or temperomandibular joint (TMJ) syndrome."

As Dr. Josephs reflected on his career, it quickly became evident that he loved what he did. "Medicine is a career in which you get to use your brain and you meet interesting people," he said. "It's an occupation in which I can make a good living and I don't ever have to sell anyone something they don't want. All I have to do is a good job, and I can be successful."

You have heard Dr. Josephs's perspective on the life of an allergist/immunologist. In the next chapter, we will discuss public health and policy.

CHAPTER 23

PUBLIC HEALTH AND PUBLIC POLICY

I interviewed two physicians, both with degrees in public health.

Dr. Susan Lovich is a pediatrician who also has a master's degree in public health. "As a student, I would have liked to know about all the different career possibilities for physicians. It is nice to know there is a world of different opportunities, even within one particular specialty. Doctors are definitely not confined only to clinical medicine." Susan's father was a doctor, but she didn't always know that she wanted to go into medicine. She pursued an undergraduate degree in applied biology, and then later, she realized that she enjoyed medicine because it combined science as well as working with people.

After completing medical school and a pediatric residency, a mentor encouraged her to get her degree in public health. "For me, this was a pathway to a leadership position," she said during our interview. "Within the field there are many opportunities, including international health, health policy, epidemiology (the study of cause, prevalence, and control of disease in populations), and biostatistics. I was interested in administration from a healthcare perspective."

I asked what advice she had for those of you considering a medical career. "Go into medicine," said Dr. Lovich, "but only if your heart is in it. It has to be a calling." She went on to state that a career in medicine provides satisfaction and stability, saying, "You may not be rich, but you will have a job."

Although Dr. Lovich currently spends most of her working time practicing clinical medicine, her background in public health has taught her about the resources available to doctors to effect change and create new policy. She explained that doctors are in a unique position to understand public health needs and make policy suggestions, but it is far more effective if done in a group. "The different medical factions like the American Medical Association and local medical societies are powerful tools for creating change," said Dr. Lovich. "The American Academy of Pediatrics, for example, has education and legislative divisions. If pediatricians want to, they can join organized medicine and become involved. It is similar for physicians in other specialties."

"If you are passionate about a cause," said Dr. Naomi Baumslag, "form your own group." She herself has earned a master's degree in public health, become President of the Women's International Public Health Network, and championed many noble causes as well. She has been a longtime advocate for maternal health, infant nutrition, and breast-feeding. "Gather other people who are like-minded and make noise," she said. "We have power in numbers."

As a doctor, one has many opportunities outside of clinical practice, including the opportunity to change and encourage change in public policy and health care.

PUBLIC HEALTH

CHAPTER 24

SURGERY

A general surgeon is a physician who specializes in the operative (surgical) treatment of diseases, injuries, and other disorders. Training involves four years of medical school followed by five to six years of residency.

What made speaking to the following two surgeons particularly interesting is that they are father and son. Although there are similarities to the way they practice, they each have their own unique perspective.

"I always equated being a doctor with being a surgeon," said Dr. Jerome L. Sandler, who completed his medical training at Jefferson in Philadelphia and then, inspired by the chief of surgery, John H. Gibbon Jr., remained there for a surgical residency. "Since high school, I knew I wanted to be a doctor," he continued. "I had an uncle who was a dermatologist. While I was in college, I visited him in his office on several occasions and became even more interested in medicine. After my first year of college, I took a job developing X rays at Doctor's Hospital and the following year, a classmate and I answered an ad and began working as night laboratory technicians at the same hospital. We learned how to do everything in the lab, including how to draw blood. I'll never forget when it was my colleague's turn to practice on me. He tied the tourniquet around my arm and inserted the needle with the syringe. As soon as blood appeared in the syringe, he became dizzy and passed out, with the needle still in my arm."

I wondered what led Dr. Sandler to choose a surgical career. "In medical school, I enjoyed everything in the clinical sciences," he said, "but I especially liked surgery." He then told me that it was a wonderful experience to work with a surgeon as brilliant as Dr. Gibbon. "I admired him very much," said Dr. Sandler. "He had a dream while at Harvard in 1933 that if you could take the blood out of the body and oxygenate it, you could bypass the heart and perform open heart surgery. In 1953, Dr. Gibbon performed the first successful open heart surgical procedure on a woman with a septal defect on total cardiopulmonary bypass. He changed the face of cardiac surgery and made it an everyday procedure."

"Some physicians may choose surgery because they desire more instant gratification," said Dr. Sandler. "A surgical career is very rewarding because patients come in requiring surgery for whatever reason and the majority go home well. However, complications can be severe, and concern for the patient can occupy you completely. At one point in my career, I contemplated becoming a pediatric surgeon, but that changed after one particularly sad case. I was a first-year resident at Jefferson, working with a pediatric surgeon who had completed nine years of residency and was completing an additional year to qualify for the thoracic surgery boards. Together, we saw a premature infant with an incarcerated hernia. Soon after surgery for the hernia, the baby developed staph (staphylococcus) pneumonia and succumbed. The pain of loss of this infant was such that I decided I could not go through that again, especially since the mortality associated with congenital anomalies in those days was so high. Today, the success rate for correction of those anomalies is laudable."

Dr. Sandler told me about another tragic situation. "A patient had empyema (presence of pus in a cavity) of the gall bladder and also had a severe heart problem. There was a debate about whether he could tolerate the surgery. We decided that we had no choice but to go ahead with the surgery. Unfortunately, in the operating room the patient had a cardiac arrest, and we pumped his chest and tried to resuscitate him until we had to give up, and he was pronounced dead.

I was the one to go out to tell the family that the patient had died. I returned to the operating room and was stunned when the cardiologist notified me that the patient's heart had resumed beating and he had a measurable blood pressure. Can you imagine having to explain this to his family? I did. Five days later, he died. That was one of the worst experiences of my career."

Dr. Sandler reminded me that despite the challenges, he has participated in many rewarding experiences. "As chief resident, I treated a thirty-nine-year-old woman who was driving with her family and was hit head-on by a car. She was brought to the emergency room with a 'flail chest.' We resuscitated her and took her to the operating room. I stuck a needle into her pericardium and got blood. When we opened her chest, I saw a tear in her atrium (heart chamber). Thankfully, we were able to sew it up, and she survived."

He then described another happy outcome to me. "A woman came in with a moon (round-swollen) face and increased facial hair. It turned out these symptoms were caused by an adrenal gland tumor and Cushing's disease. I operated on her and removed the tumor. On the final follow-up visit, her husband gave me a hug and said, 'Thank you for giving me my beautiful wife back.'

"There were unusual experiences, too," said Dr. Sandler. "When I was chief resident, a member of the mafia was shot and injured badly. I operated on him, and he thanked me by giving me a book on how to appreciate wine. The salary for residents in those days was $100 per month. In the book, there were five crisp, new $100 bills—five months' wages."

Jerome Sandler is a highly respected surgeon, a member of the American College of Surgeons, and has had a remarkable career. As I spoke to him, I got the impression that more than any of his own accomplishments, he is most proud of his son, Glenn, who is also a surgeon and who joined him as a partner in his office. Of course, I asked what it was like to work with his own son. "It's fabulous," he said. "A week after he started working with me, a doctor called to refer him a patient with her seventh bout of intestinal obstruction. My son called me and asked if I would give him a hand because this was going to be a difficult case. I was happy to do so but wondered how I could impart my pearls of wisdom without insulting him. He started operating and I soon realized I didn't have to open my mouth. He knew exactly what he was doing and did it beautifully. Every once in a while—when we would do a case together—that was a wonderful experience, since it almost seemed there was a genetic similarity in how we operated and anticipated each other's movements."

"If you want to become a surgeon," said Dr. Glenn Sandler, "you must be able to endure an intense training period during which you will have to make difficult decisions in a variety of circumstances. As a surgeon, you also need to be able to accept some degree of uncertainty." Both his father and uncle are surgeons, so Glenn had exposure to the medical field growing up. "You have to pick a career you think you will enjoy," he said, "and I enjoy what I do—taking care of people and being constantly challenged."

"About three months ago, I operated on a patient with a large spleen the size of a basketball," said Dr. Sandler. "His spleen occupied most of his abdominal space. At the very moment that I was going to ligate (tie off) the splenic artery and vein, the patient started to bleed from the splenic vein. There was rapid bleeding, and I couldn't apply effective pressure due to the size of the spleen. I knew that the patient could die in thirty seconds if I did nothing; there was no time to waste. I didn't have many options and instinctively pulled his spleen out of his body while at the same time holding pressure over the blood vessels to stop the bleeding. Thankfully, in this case, the maneuver turned out to be the right thing to do, and I was able to sew up the vein, and the patient recovered without incident." Dr. Sandler will never forget that day. "Preserving life is the most rewarding aspect of medicine."

He has endured some very difficult experiences, too. One of his longstanding patients was diagnosed with cancer and subsequently had a recurrence. He has taken care of her every step of the way. "She is one of my favorite patients," he said, "but there are times when the diseases we treat evade our therapies despite our best efforts."

Dr. Sandler obtained his medical degree from the University of Maryland and then completed his surgical residency at Albert Einstein in Philadelphia. His numerous accomplishments included serving as chief of surgery at Shady Grove Hospital in Maryland and building a surgical center where he currently operates on most of his patients. He also mentors students and takes them on clinical rounds. "I like what I do, and I don't find this job too stressful," he said, "although I think that is more a reflection of one's internal makeup than of a surgical career per se."

Now, you have heard from two surgeons who graduated from medical school a generation apart. In the next chapter, Dr. Stark and Dr. Lieberman will each speak about the field of psychiatry.

CHAPTER 25

PSYCHIATRY

A psychiatrist is a physician who is a specialist in the treatment of mental and emotional disorders. Psychiatrists are medical doctors and are licensed to prescribe medication. Training includes four years of medical school followed by a psychiatry residency.

DR. STARK'S POINT OF VIEW

"I believe it is most important to take a careful history and conduct a good clinical exam and rely on your experience and judgment rather than have the lab diagnose. The psychological tests are there to address questions the clinician has. To be a fine clinician is critical, and that differentiates the good doctor from the mediocre," said Dr. William Stark, commenting on the makings of an above-average doctor.

Dr. Stark obtained his medical degree in 1943 and then completed his residency training in neurology and psychiatry at Albany Hospital in Albany, New York. He completed a tour of active duty with the U.S. Navy, serving as chief of psychiatry at the U.S. Naval Hospital in Jacksonville, Florida.

He received his fellowship training in neuropathology and neurology at the George Washington University Hospital and then in child psychiatry at the University Hospital in Baltimore, Maryland. In addition to being certified in adult, child, and adolescent psychiatry, Dr. Stark is also certified in psychoanalysis, and child and adolescent psychoanalysis.

In 1950, he opened a private practice and soon after joined the faculty at George Washington University as a clinical professor of psychiatry and behavioral sciences and pediatrics. Dr. Stark served as the first director of the division of adolescent psychiatry at Children's National Medical Center and also served as a consultant to other institutions, including the National Institute of Mental Health. In addition, he was the first president of the Washington Council of Child and Adolescent Psychiatry and the treasurer of the American Academy of Child and Adolescent Psychiatry.

Dr. Stark has held a number of academic positions and has been a pioneer in the field of child and adolescent psychiatry. For his leadership, service, and outstanding contributions to the field, he was granted the status of Clinical Professor Emeritus at George Washington University Medical Center.

At the time of my interview with Dr. Stark, he had been practicing psychiatry in the Washington metropolitan area for fifty-seven years. Still, one patient in particular really stood out in his mind, a five-year-old autistic child who was referred to him. At that time, children with autism were usually treated in institutions, so it was not common for them to be seen in private practice. He doesn't know what made him take on this responsibility, but he wanted to help the child. The young boy wouldn't speak but would roll around on the floor making sounds. Because he was noncommunicative and would avoid any eye contact, Dr. Stark tried to engage him by imitating his behavior and sounds, hoping he would take cognizance of his presence. He met with him regularly, several times a week, and after about eighteen months, a remarkable breakthrough occurred. The office had an air conditioner in the window, and on that particular day, the young boy pointed to the unit and uttered his very first words: "air conditioner." Ultimately, after about two and a half years, he was able to attend a special school.

"One thing that intrigued me at the time was the management of emotionally disturbed children in the classroom," Dr. Stark said. He became involved in a research project at a local school to integrate the emotionally disturbed child into the normal classroom. He is understandably happy with the progress over the years; good facilities and residential treatment centers are now available for emotionally disturbed children, whereas there were minimal if any resources in the past.

I wanted to hear a psychiatrist's opinions on practicing in the twenty-first century, and when I inquired, Dr. Stark was quite definite. "I have been fortunate in the sense that I never got caught up in the managed care system. It is an impossible situation." He went on to state that because of the restrictions managed care imposes, it can compromise what physicians can do, in addition to dictating how much time is spent with patients and which costs will be covered. "Medicine has become more of a business than a profession unto itself," he added.

Some of Dr. Stark's happiest moments occurred when he taught medical students and fellows. He conducted conferences on counter-transference, which refers to aspects of the therapist's feelings and responses that may interfere with the treatment of the patient. He explained that individual psychotherapy is a two-person engagement. The conferences focused on examining what exactly was happening with the therapist during the therapeutic hour in order to help the therapist better understand his patient.

When I asked Dr. Stark what led him to enter the field of medicine, he told me that he admired doctors as a young child and was inspired when reading about people in medicine and science. "The fact that my parents encouraged me in that direction was helpful. In those days, the physician was looked upon as a respected individual." He then informed me that in the 1930s and 1940s, there was actually a quota, and only a limited number of Jewish students were accepted into medical school. Being Jewish himself, he did not take his acceptance lightly when he was accepted.

Dr. Stark said one of the biggest challenges as a psychiatrist is connecting with the patient and trying to really understand what the issues are, especially in the case of children who don't communicate well. "Also, one has to learn to separate one's issues from the patient's issues. In other words, it is important to empathize without identifying with the patient."

Finally, I asked him if he had any more words of wisdom for students interested in a career in psychiatry. "Yes, and this may be disillusioning to young physicians starting out," Dr. Stark said. "We have to learn as physicians that we are not omnipotent, and we can't cure everything. We can always maintain hope and not give up, but we should recognize our limits. I do believe that certain people are more suited to the field. As a psychiatrist, you need to be able to deal with people, be well-balanced, and really understand humanity. Although the practice of medicine is very different—and in many ways more difficult today than what it was decades ago—if you really want to become a doctor, you should follow your dream. Don't be discouraged."

I was fortunate to be able to interview a second psychiatrist so that you could have greater insight into the field. As with other medical specialties, psychiatry is broad, and there is definite variation in the type of practices and lifestyles among psychiatrists.

DR. LIEBERMAN'S POINT OF VIEW

Psychiatrist Dr. E. James Lieberman doesn't remember being passionate about becoming a doctor as a young child, but his father was an internist, and growing up watching him practice medicine made Dr. Lieberman believe that becoming a doctor would be a good accomplishment.

During medical school, he enjoyed his psychiatry rotation. "Starting in the second year, you could see a patient with supervision for one hour a week," he said. "The idea was not to make you into a psychiatrist, but rather to make you into an understanding physician. I became interested in doing psychotherapy because I had a wonderful supervisor." Dr. Lieberman said this mentor had faith in his abilities and helped him develop confidence, a personality trait he didn't always demonstrate. He remembers his first clinic patient, a woman in her fifties with an anxiety disorder. Unfortunately. the medical student–patient relationship didn't last very long. "After about four weeks, the patient informed me that she was going to pursue alternative treatment in the form of 'science of mind,' as she thought I was as anxious as she was. She was right."

His second patient was a younger woman in her mid-thirties. He remembers her looking at him and saying, "What does a doctor like you know about life? Aren't you kind of young to be dealing with these issues?" It turned out that she was having an affair with a married man whose wife was about to give birth to their third child. The supervisor, who was present for the initial session, interjected, "Dr. Lieberman is a good listener. What may be hardest for you is to hear what you have to say yourself." This helped give Dr. Lieberman the confidence to continue. The patient attended weekly sessions for six months and improved considerably. Dr. Lieberman became increasingly motivated to enter the field of psychiatry.

"I was in a dilemma during my senior year because I was then undecided about whether to go into psychiatry or preventive medicine," Dr. Lieberman told me. "I then heard a lecture by Dr. Brock Chisholm, the first director of the WHO (World Health Organization), a Canadian psychiatrist, who said you could do both. Psychiatrists could have a public health orientation." Dr. Lieberman's internship happened to be with the public health service, and during that year, he became convinced that he wanted to enter the field of psychiatry. His third year of residency was spent in a child clinic, and that experience helped foster his interest in families. He spent seven years at the National Institute of Mental Health (NIMH) in community mental health before going into private practice and teaching. He also consulted on issues of preventive psychiatry, including marriage counseling, sex education, and family planning.

He firmly believes it is very important that you like people if you want to become a psychiatrist. "You also have to be able to tolerate uncertainty. You go into every consultation knowing that you will never fully understand this person or yourself. At the present time, physicians are trained to label people with a diagnosis, mostly for insurance purposes." Dr. Lieberman went on to say that this practice supposedly enables the practitioner to decide which form of treatment and which medication to use—a convenient reasoning—but psychiatrists should avoid locking themselves into a diagnosis that could prove erroneous or proposed too soon. "A philosophical orientation is good. Each individual is unique. In a way, psychiatrists are practicing philosophy as well as science."

When I asked him if he thought doctors would soon have better chemical or biological markers for psychiatric diagnoses, he replied, "I don't think we will ever fully explain humans with chemistry, although we will learn a lot more about brain function." Additionally, Dr. Lieberman took a course on hypnosis and said that he gained much from that study. "We're always involved in inadvertent suggestion. The hypnotist is tuned in to how we sound when we talk. It's not enough to have the right diagnosis and interpretation or suggestion; it has to be stated in the right way. We have to be self-aware so the patient feels we are accurately empathic, not just sympathetic."

I wanted to know what difficulties and challenges psychiatrists face and whether they take their patients' problems home with them. Dr. Lieberman said that he does at times. "A particular worry is a patient who doesn't show up for an appointment and does not call," he mentioned. Once, one of his patients didn't show up for an appointment, and Dr. Lieberman soon found out that this patient had taken an overdose and was rushed to the emergency room. In another challenging case, Dr. Lieberman remembers being on the phone with a patient who called him after hours and sounded hysterical. She said that she was in the living room, and through her window, she could see a man outside. She sounded so afraid it didn't occur to him this was not true, that it was a conscious falsehood dramatized to test him. "A common difficulty is ending a therapy session when dealing with challenging and frustrating issues. The ability to separate is very important, and it's tough. Usually, it's better to schedule an extra session than to prolong a regular one."

Finally, reflecting on his career, Dr. Lieberman added, "Of course, the most difficult thing to deal with is a patient's suicide. Almost every psychiatrist has at least one suicide and several close calls."

CHAPTER 26

EMERGENCY ROOM MEDICINE

Emergency room physicians are doctors who specialize in the care of patients with urgent or life-threatening conditions. Training includes four years of medical school followed by a three- or four-year residency.

Dr. Julian Orenstein told me that he initially went into medicine to please his father rather than to fulfill a childhood dream. His dad, a Holocaust survivor, was a general practitioner who wanted his sons to become doctors. Because his oldest brother didn't follow a medical path, Dr. Orenstein felt obligated to do so. He majored in biology at the University of Pennsylvania and then was accepted into medical school at Syracuse. At that point, there was no turning back. Dr. Orenstein found that medical school was more challenging for him because he had not taken college-level anatomy and physiology courses. Whereas this material was easier for some of the other students, much of it was new for him. Naturally, he began to have doubts about whether or not he was doing the right thing, but as his career progressed, he became more satisfied with his choice.

In medical school, Dr. Orenstein spent much of the first year dissecting a cadaver, and he found this to be one of his most difficult times. The rest of the first two years were mainly spent doing classroom work, but later on, when he had more exposure to direct patient care, he realized that he had made the right decision after all. On another note, Dr. Orenstein had always wanted to write, and he did so during college as well as medical school. He wrote articles on the satisfaction of caring for patients that appeared in newspapers and online magazines, and he also authored scientific articles and a series of three books.

Once Dr. Orenstein graduated from medical school, he completed a three-year pediatric residency as well as a two-year fellowship program. Since then, he has been practicing emergency room medicine in the Washington metropolitan area.

During our interview, I asked Dr. Orenstein about the highlights and the difficulties he has faced in his career over the years. He described how difficult it was when he was confronted with a critically ill child, and when he recognized that a patient had an illness such as a malignancy and their prognosis would be poor. "You have to reassure them that there are tests to be done and there is treatment they can pursue. There are so many stressful situations one faces in the emergency room. I find that my team makes a big difference. It's not so much an issue about whether I've worked with them before, but more about how much experience they've had. Sometimes a temp nurse can be excellent. The satisfying times are when everything runs smoothly and when a critically ill or dying baby can be brought back and given another chance to live. There's nothing like seeing the heart monitor spring back to life."

As an emergency room physician you will be responsible for evaluating and treating patients with acute illnesses and injuries, and will likely perform numerous procedures such as lumbar punctures, intubation, cardiopulmonary resuscitation and more.

In this section, Dr. Orenstein revealed what motivated him to become a doctor and described a few of the challenges that emergency room physicians face. In the next chapter, Dr. Silverberg will talk about the field of pathology.

CHAPTER 27

PATHOLOGY

A pathologist is a physician who is an expert in laboratory medicine as well as the analysis of body cells, tissues, fluids, and other specimens in order to make a diagnosis. Training involves the completion of four years of medical school followed by a residency in pathology and sometimes a fellowship.

"I remember the exact moment I decided to become a pathologist," said Dr. Marc Silverberg. "Do you remember the concept of roundsmanship?" he asked me. I thought back to my time in medical school and remembered the hierarchy on clinical rounds. Medical students were made to feel rather insignificant at times, and the attendings were treated like gods. "It's something like that," he told me and then started into his story. "I was doing my surgery rotation in medical school at Yale. In the operating room, surgical specimens were couriered to the pathology lab by medical students who had to wait for a reading and then bring back a slip with a preliminary diagnosis. I remember how the specimen used to disappear and then how an answer would return. The chief pathology resident and the pathology attending, a former marine who could probably eat residents for breakfast, would sit together, looking at the slide through a double-headed scope. The pressure was on. I remember the attending going, "Hmmm," and then, peering into the eyes of the chief resident, he asked, 'Well, what do *you* think it is?' The resident peered back into the attending's eyes. 'I don't know.' *Oh, never say that*, I thought.

I had been taught to give an answer always. The resident continued with, 'What do you think it is?' I was surprised he had the audacity to speak to an attending that way. I was mesmerized and wondered what would happen next. The attending's eyes narrowed, and his face tightened, and then he said calmly, 'I don't know either. Let's look it up!' I couldn't believe my ears. I thought to myself, 'Wait a minute. They're not trying to compete? Their only concern is finding the right diagnosis for the patient?' That's the moment I knew pathology was the field for me."

Dr. Silverberg's father was (and still is) a cardiologist, and Dr. Silverberg remembers accompanying him to a hospital in Washington, D.C., after which his father would take him to Chinatown. He enjoyed those trips, and, Dr. Silverberg said to me as he laughed, for a while he associated becoming a doctor with eating Chinese food. He briefly considered the possibility of following in his dad's footsteps but pursued a career in music instead. Dr. Silverberg graduated from the Curtis Institute in Philadelphia and then changed paths later in life. He completed a second undergraduate degree at George Washington University in Washington, D.C., before going to medical school at Yale. After medical school, he completed a residency in pathology and then a one-year fellowship in oncologic pathology.

Dr. Silverberg is currently a successful pathologist, and the owner and director of a large practice in Norfolk, Virginia. I asked him to briefly describe the life of a pathologist for readers. "People often think of a pathologist as being someone isolated in a lab—perhaps in the basement of a hospital. On the contrary, although I don't have much direct patient contact, I interact with almost every other physician in the hospital all the time. We also know what goes on with many of the patients in the hospital, because most of them have some lab interaction."

Enthusiastically, he then explained that pathology is an exciting field. "I was always someone who had curiosity and wanted to find answers. Pathology is a field that allows one to search for answers. For me it's still about solving the puzzle, and that's what keeps me going. However, you must be comfortable with the fact that you will not find the answers to everything." Next, he told me that pathologists see something they've never seen before almost on a daily basis. "Common diseases sometimes manifest atypically," he continued. "Making the right diagnosis is still a great source of pride for us, and we're challenged every day. We are often viewed as providing support to other physicians, although by analyzing tissues and microscopic architecture, we frequently help to guide treatment." He added that it was ironic, however, that in his previous career, his role was that of a support musician in an orchestra.

The most challenging part of his job, Dr. Silverberg said, is adjusting to the changing role of the pathologist. In the past, he was the one to make the tissue diagnosis and provide those answers to the patient's physician, who in turn incorporated it into his or her other information. Now, it is more often the pathologist who incorporates all the diverse lab findings, analyzes them, and reports them back to the physician in a succinct summary. "The entire field of pathology has changed as we move towards best-practice, evidence-based medicine rather than basing diagnoses on one doctor's experience," he said. "There is also a drive towards personalized medicine, which involves the way patients may respond to various treatment modalities. By identifying nonresponders, we can prevent patients from getting expensive treatments that would delay their proper therapy."

I asked Dr. Silverberg if it was easy to balance his work and private life. "My hours are very good because I only have to take weekend call every fifth week," he admitted. "However, my job as a pathologist is to look for bad things and, when I find them, to keep looking for more. Can you imagine living with someone who does that?"

Dr. Silverberg has pointed out how the field of pathology has evolved and has given us an in-depth view of the life of a pathologist. In the next chapter, you'll learn more about the fields of hematology and oncology.

CHAPTER 28

HEMATOLOGY/
ONCOLOGY

A hematologist-oncologist is a physician who specializes in both hematology and oncology. A hematologist is a specialist in the diagnosis and
treatment of disorders of the blood and bone marrow, and an oncologist
is a specialist in the diagnosis and treatment of cancers.

Dr. Alla Shapiro is a pediatric hematologist-oncologist who is also
a medical officer in the Office of Counterterrorism and Emergency
Coordination at the Food and Drug Administration (FDA). She obtained
her medical degree and a PhD in the Ukraine, where she later specialized
in pediatric hematology. Her mother was a physician and strongly influenced her decision to enter into medicine. "I knew I would be a doctor
when I was five years old," said Dr. Shapiro. In 1986, however, she was not
prepared to become one of the first responders in the Chernobyl disaster,
the worst nuclear power plant accident in history. But being a hematologist and living only 60 miles away from the site qualified her for the job.
What Dr. Shapiro saw there was chaos and tragedy, which only fueled her
passion to find something to protect people against radiation exposure.
"When the rescue workers walked barefoot just a short distance to save
the victims, they returned with burns on their feet and legs that looked
like red socks. I'll never forget it," she told me during the interview.

In the United States, Dr. Shapiro completed a three-year residency
in pediatrics at Georgetown University Hospital, followed by a fellowship at the National Cancer Institute (Pediatric Branch) at the National

Institutes of Health. In her second year, she came upon an exciting discovery that would change her career path dramatically. Dr. Shapiro became a co-inventor for a drug that is expected to deliver in humans a protective or therapeutic effect against lethal radiation exposure. Being developed as a medical radiation countermeasure, this product is intended for use in the event of (or threat of) a radiation or nuclear event caused by terrorism or other nuclear accidents. I learned that currently, there are no approved drugs for use as medical radiation countermeasures for the prevention or treatment of acute radiation syndrome.

"Until then, I didn't consider medical career possibilities other than direct patient care," she said. "I rotated through the division of oncology at the FDA for two months and knew this was what interested me; so after completing my fellowship, I formally applied to the FDA." Dr. Shapiro worked in the division of oncology in the field of brain cancer for several years, and then after the terrorist attack on the United States on September 11, 2001, everything changed. Increased emphasis was placed on protecting Americans in the case of another attack. Medical countermeasures against biologic, nuclear, and chemical exposure were scarce or nonexistent. By chance one day, she opened an email from the FDA, which read that they were trying to recruit a doctor for a new division, the division of counterterrorism. She was hired for the job.

Dr. Shapiro is currently involved in several working groups, one of which estimates the needs of blood products in case of a massive explosion of a nuclear device. She also advises pharmaceutical biotech and private companies in order to help develop drugs and vaccines to protect the American public against radiation exposure. Dr. Shapiro has never doubted her career choice, but she never would have predicted the exciting path it took.

CHAPTER 29

PEDIATRICS

A pediatrician is a physician who is a specialist in the treatment of infants, children, and adolescents. Training to become a pediatrician includes four years of medical school followed by a residency of at least three years in pediatrics.

Of the following two pediatricians—Dr. Crim and later Dr. Koomson—one completed her medical school and residency training in the United States, and the other attended medical school in Ghana, and then completed a residency and fellowship in Canada before moving to the United States to practice pediatrics and emergency room medicine.

"Children are somewhat helpless and need someone to look out for them," said Dr. Lisa Crim, a pediatrician and partner in a private medical practice. "It's really fun to watch them grow up. They want to share their family experiences with me, and to some extent, I feel as if I'm part of their extended family." She recalled a recent visit with a little girl who was brought in by her mother. The daughter had just been to the hairdresser, and the mother said to Dr. Crim, "She had her hair cut just like yours."

The life of a pediatrician can be very busy, too. "We have so many patients to see that there is very little time to make follow-up phone calls during the day," said Dr. Crim, "so I usually have to do them at night. In part, I do this to myself because I encourage patients to call me with updates. I feel torn at times, balancing my needs and the needs of my patients and my family. Unlike some other jobs, when one doesn't feel well, you can't simply call in sick. I would feel as if I'm letting people down—my colleagues and my patients." Then, she told me how she makes it all work. "I find balance by working three to four days a week so that I have more time for my family and my hobbies."

Next, I asked if any experiences stood out in her mind. "Any time you save a life, you will always remember it," she said. "I saw a fifteen-month-old new patient for a routine checkup. He was screaming. I was surprised that his heart rate was so slow for a crying baby and had the sense that something was wrong. I kept listening, trying to calm the baby down, and then had to explain to the father that there may be a problem with his baby's heart. I referred them straight to a cardiologist who diagnosed a complete heart block, requiring medications and a pacemaker. The cardiologist told me, if this had not been detected, the baby could have died in his sleep. One always hopes in one's medical career that one can really make a difference. Every time I see that child I think, 'For you, my friend, I made a difference.'"

Dr. Crim started off studying music at the Peabody Conservatory in Baltimore, but after a semester, she realized that music was not the career she wanted to pursue. She switched to George Washington University to study science and music; then she completed her medical training at the University of Cincinnati and her residency at Georgetown University. "I always loved children," she said. "They're so innocent, with no baggage and no preconceived ideas. I was a nanny and frequently babysat before I started medical school. In children, you have a captive audience."

For those of you considering a career in pediatrics, Dr. Crim gave this advice: "You can't go into pediatrics thinking you're going to make a fortune, but it's certainly a rewarding and interesting job. You also need to have a sense of humor, because if you don't find the humor, you won't enjoy the work. Families usually appreciate when you try to make their kids happy, and the kids often have funny things to say. You must have patience and give people the time they need. My patients understand when I sometimes run late. They know it's not because I'm in the back playing tiddlywinks or eating bon-bons." From her words and dedication, I could tell how much this pediatrician cared about her patients. "In this field, you can't easily leave everything at the office at the end of the day," she said. "One thinks about the patients and worries about them because they're all so vulnerable."

PEDIATRICS—ANOTHER POINT OF VIEW

"I've always liked working with children," said pediatrician Dr. Bertha Koomson, "because they're fun. They also get better faster, and once they do, they generally remain healthy."

Bertha's father was a doctor, and even as a little girl, she knew she wanted to follow in his footsteps. "I've always been high-achieving, and I thought I should be able to do whatever I wanted, even though I was a woman," she said. "I grew up and attended medical school in Ghana where only about 10 percent of my class was female. It made me work that much harder." She then told me that medical school was rigorous. "You're expected to know a lot and do a lot. You only appreciate the hard work and what you've learned later. In residency, I first realized that what I had learned in medical school I could put into practice. At this point in my life when certain knowledge comes to me naturally, it's also thanks to my medical school training."

After medical school, Dr. Koomson worked as a general practitioner in Ghana for a year, and then went to Canada to complete a pediatric residency and a fellowship in pediatric emergency medicine. She later moved to the United States and is currently working in a private pediatric practice, although she occasionally does shifts in a local pediatric emergency department.

Next, she spoke about one of the challenges of practicing pediatrics in this decade. "Patients are able to access medical information online and are often very well-informed," she said. "They come in with certain expectations, and as a pediatrician, one has to be prepared to discuss their concerns in a way that is logical to them. For example, a patient's mother told me that her child had a rash. She went online and read about hand, foot, and mouth disease, then called to tell me that was what he had. I had to explain to her that in order for me to make a diagnosis, it was best that I looked at the rash myself. Another issue that arises is concern about the perceived dangers of immunizations. I often have to convince parents that immunizations are still generally safe."

Dr. Koomson told me that if she had to start over, she would definitely choose pediatrics again. To those of you interested in becoming pediatricians, she recommended that you take into consideration what type of lifestyle and reward you want. "In most cases, pediatrics will involve taking calls, and it can be very busy. Pediatricians, including those in private practice, also usually spend some of their time doing hospital rounds, whether that may be checking newborns or taking care of sick patients. We are not the best paid specialists, but there are other rewards. You get to know the families and watch the kids grow up. I haven't seen many unhappy pediatricians; most love what they do. There have also been exciting advances in the field. Since we began the routine use of the HIB (hemophilus influenza bacterium) vaccine, we have seen fewer serious illnesses caused by this infection, and the pneumococcal vaccine has reduced the incidence of middle ear infections. Another example is the progress that has been made in prenatal diagnosis. Now, undiagnosed cardiac problems have become a rarity in the United States."

Finally, I asked Dr. Koomson what type of personality might be more suited to a pediatric career. "All types of personalities choose pediatrics," she said. "You will develop your personality and your own style as you go along, but—most importantly—you have to like kids. Speaking as a pediatrician who is a mother, I think one's own children give you a different perspective." That said, she also believes that perspective is shared by pediatricians who are fathers. "As a parent, it is also challenging

PEDIATRICS

to balance work and family time. There's a certain way of life that you become accustomed to—for example, taking calls and working late. Don't expect to be done at five. However, it is also a great profession, and a job you can always do wherever you are, until you retire."

In this section, you heard from two pediatricians with very different medical backgrounds and experiences. Now, read the next chapter and hear from an orthopedist.

CHAPTER 30

ORTHOPEDICS AND SPORTS MEDICINE

An orthopedic surgeon (orthopedist) is a physician who specializes in the treatment of injuries and disorders of the musculoskeletal system. Training includes four years of medical school usually followed by at least five years of residency.

"My family used to say, 'They can take away your clothes, but they can't take away what's between your ears,'" said Dr. Richard Reff, a pediatric orthopedic surgeon and specialist in sports medicine for adults and children.

"There was always a reverence for doctors. My grandfather was an immigrant from Russia and came to the United States when he was sixteen. My grandmother came to America from the Ukraine to go to medical school but was unable to do so because circumstances arose whereupon the doors weren't open to her. In 1913 and 1914, women weren't given a lot of opportunities," said Dr. Reff.

He went on to say that even when he was a boy—once he became less scared of getting shots from the pediatrician—he became very taken by physicians and held them in high regard. "In high school, I gravitated to the sciences because I was interested, but also because I knew that one had to excel in those subjects to be a doctor. My other real passion was sports, but at that time, I had no idea that I could combine the two into a career."

Towards the end of college and the beginning of medical school at George Washington University, Dr. Reff became friendly with an orthopedist who was involved with a sports team. "He invited me to the football games at the University of Maryland, and it looked exciting to me," he said. "I got a chance to see firsthand what a doctor in the field was doing. During medical school, I knew that I was ready to be a surgeon. I had an interest from day one in the anatomy lab. I had no problem with dissection. At George Washington, we had some marvelous teachers, including the editor of *Gray's Anatomy*, Dr. Charles Mayo Goss. He was so inspiring. We also had an anatomy professor from Walter Reed Army Hospital. When it came to the extremities of the cadaver, he would do the dissections, and we would learn from him. In my third year of medical school during my pediatrics rotation, I did my project on Little Leaguer's elbow. I was gravitating towards orthopedics."

He told me the beginning of his career was as a pediatric orthopedic surgeon at Children's Hospital in Washington, D.C., and then later, he expanded to include sports medicine. Today, his office walls are adorned with photographs inscribed with thanks from basketball players, ballerinas, gymnasts, and other athletes. Dr. Reff also acts as a consultant to student health services at the University of Maryland. During our interview, he spoke about some of the advances in the field. "Television has changed the way physicians look at sports and injuries. With slow-motion technology a doctor can look at the way an injury is happening." This technology, he told me, not only helps us understand the mechanism itself but may also help us prevent future injuries.

Students interested in a career in orthopedics have several options. Some orthopedists spend most of their time in the office seeing patients, while others may prefer doing procedures such as spinal and reconstructive surgery or super-specializing in specific anatomy areas such as the shoulder. Though Dr. Reff didn't name any specific character traits essential to those interested in this career, he strongly felt that they should have an aptitude for physics, biomechanics, and spatial relationships.

Next, Dr. Reff spoke about managed care and the difficulties of being in practice. "Over the last several years, it costs more money to operate

ORTHOPEDICS

an office, and you receive less money for the services you provide, so there is more pressure to pay the overhead. The business side of medicine can't be ignored."

But would he still choose the same career if he could start all over? "I would still do it," he stated. "Medicine has afforded me the opportunity to do things that I could not otherwise have done. For example, during my residency, I spent six months in New Zealand. I worked as a doctor at the Atlanta Olympics and have been involved in the U.S. Olympic Committee."

Finally, I asked if he had any words of advice or encouragement for students. Without hesitation, he left me with these words: "Medicine is still a very admirable and respected profession in which you can help a lot of people. There is so much fulfillment from thanks that doesn't have a price tag on it."

You have now read about a number of physicians in clinical practice. Some doctors are interested in the research aspect of medicine; others may want to combine clinical medicine and research. Next, we will hear from two physician-scientists.

CHAPTER 31

PHYSICIAN-SCIENTISTS— RESEARCH

Physician-scientists (research physicians) are doctors who have undergone training in both medicine and research. While these professionals usually spend most of their time doing research, they also teach and practice clinical medicine quite frequently. They are involved in work that has the potential to advance our knowledge and understanding of science and disease, which ultimately leads to groundbreaking new treatments. For example, Dr. Arthur Kornberg was awarded the Nobel Prize in medicine for his work on DNA. Physician-scientists usually find positions at research institutions, within the pharmaceutical industry, or sometimes on the faculty of universities or medical centers.

You may pursue various pathways towards a career in medical research. Today, most students interested in becoming physician-scientists pursue an MD/PhD degree, although some students complete their medical training first and then enter into the research field. Thankfully, a large number of medical schools in the United States now offer MD/PhD programs. For more information on these programs, visit the AAMC website at www.aamc.com.

Now that you understand the basics of the physician-scientist profession, listen to the following perspectives of two different doctors.

DR. MITCHELL MAX

"There is an explosion of molecular science, which could potentially treat disease, but unfortunately a shortage of MDs who can apply this understanding clinically," said Dr. Mitchell Max.

Dr. Max, a visiting professor of anesthesiology and medicine as well as the director of the Molecular Epidemiology of Pain Program at the University of Pittsburgh, described his fascinating research, which culminated in the discovery of three genes that affect people's perception of pain. Listening to Dr. Max describe his pioneering work, one might think the field of research would be limited to a select few individuals, but he interjected, "Somebody who has the intellectual ability to get through medical school and become a competent physician has what it takes to become a clinical researcher."

There are various pathways that you can pursue should you wish to enter the field of research. For example, you may pursue an MD/PhD degree or complete a master's in public health. After graduating from Harvard Medical School, Dr. Max completed three years of internal medicine and three years of neurology before beginning his clinical research. Whatever he did, he always found himself looking for more answers—in his case, more choices for treating and dealing with pain. The answers were not initially obvious, so he had to find them. As a result of his ambition, he became director of the pain clinic at the National Institutes of Health (NIH) and a world-renowned expert on the genetic basis of pain.

He has found his career to be very rewarding intellectually, and it has also afforded him financial security. Dr. Max also described the challenges facing physicians in the research field. One common difficulty faced by researchers is obtaining funding for studies; another is dealing with the logistics of clinical trials, which includes concerns about safety, the avoidance of side effects, and minimizing the dropout rate.

His advice to physicians going into the research field is to find good mentorship, choose an institution that really cares about research, and pick an important problem to study. Most programs will guarantee mentorship for the first few years—for example, in the form of a training grant—and thereafter, one becomes an independent researcher.

DR. ROSCOE BRADY

"Know that this work is time-consuming. Have lots of patience, but consider giving yourself a time limit for making a significant discovery," is Dr. Roscoe Brady's advice to students interested in research.

Dr. Brady was chief of the Developmental and Metabolic Branch of the National Institute of Neurological Disorders and Stroke at the NIH. At the time of our interview, he was Scientist Emeritus at the NIH. As I spoke to him, it was difficult not to be awestruck by this man. After all, he was responsible for much groundbreaking research, including the discovery of the cause as well as the treatment of Gaucher disease, the most prevalent hereditary metabolic storage disorder of humans.

Dr. Brady received his MD from Harvard Medical School and interned at the Hospital of the University of Pennsylvania. He did a postdoctoral fellowship in the department of biochemistry at the University of Pennsylvania as well. He has received numerous awards, including the Albert Lasker Award for Clinical Medical Research and the U.S. National Medal of Technology and Innovation. He is a member of the National Academy of Sciences (NAS) and the Institute of Medicine of the NAS. Dr. Brady's branch investigates hereditary diseases and develops treatments for patients with these conditions.

In his second semester of medical school, Dr. Brady worked with a professor researching alcoholism in rats. They knew that if you took away B vitamins, the rats drank more alcohol. They discovered that the rats decreased their alcohol consumption for a time when they were given vitamin B but quickly reverted to drinking large quantities even while receiving the vitamin. This indicated that some changes had occurred in the animals consuming alcohol that were more complex than simple vitamin deficiencies. Although the research turned out well, he learned how time-consuming it could be, and he only completed the project in his last semester of medical school. One payoff was that he received the prize for the best medical student research in his fourth year, and perhaps this motivated him to continue a career in research.

During his third year of medical school, he became deeply affected when a twenty-six-year-old patient died of heart disease. Another significant loss occurred in his fourth year when a patient died while undergoing cardiac bypass surgery. He knew that there was so much more that needed to be understood and done. Dr. Brady had decided on his path but gave himself a time limit to pursue research. The first postdoctoral year at the University of Pennsylvania was very difficult and unproductive; only later did it become better. During his third year, he discovered the enzyme complex that produced long-chain fatty acids. After his fourth year, however, he was called to active duty in the U.S. Navy and so could not continue this research. Naturally, this frustrated him, but he did what he could, working in a laboratory at the NIH at night.

After two and a half years, he was asked to join NIH to research lipid material in nerves and better understand the cause of multiple sclerosis. This led him to his groundbreaking work on Gaucher, Niemann-Pick, Fabry, and Tay-Sachs diseases. Prior to his research, nothing was known about the metabolism of the accumulating substances and which (if any) enzymes might be underactive in the various disorders. In each case, these patients are missing a key enzyme, without which toxic materials accumulate throughout the body, including the brain in many cases. After many years of additional work, Dr. Brady developed his successful enzyme replacement treatment for patients with Gaucher disease, the most prevalent of these disorders. Patients now live normal lives with a brief intravenous infusion of the missing enzyme every two weeks. Dr. Brady is one of two people who discovered the cause of a disease and also developed a highly successful treatment for it.

At this point, I started to wonder if there were any noticeable character traits that might identify future researchers, and toward the end of our interview, I discovered that Dr. Brady loved organic chemistry. How many medical students can honestly say that?

CHAPTER 32

MY OWN REFLECTIONS

Having spoken to a vast number of physicians and interviewed several, I find I have even more faith in the medical profession than before. The doctors I interviewed went into medicine for the right reasons and seemed to care deeply for their patients and their craft. They each spoke of the satisfaction one derives from helping others. They also illustrated the many opportunities available to those in the medical profession. Although most seemed happy with their decisions to enter their fields, they did point out the negative aspects as well, including the long hours and the hassles of dealing with managed care companies.

After each interview, however, I emerged with a greater understanding of the medical profession and more insight into my own career and feelings about medicine. They were all kind enough to let me (and my readers) into their worlds and share their struggles and their triumphs.

In summation, I have enjoyed writing this book and am grateful to all the students, doctors, and other experts who have made it possible. I hope that you have been inspired by the stories you have read and now know the steps you should take in order to pursue your goals. If you remain passionate about becoming a doctor, I am confident that you will achieve your dream and will undoubtedly contribute to making a positive difference in this world.

PART THREE

REVIEW AND
RESOURCES

In the next section you will find answers to frequently asked questions, a guide to the medical school application process, information on international medical graduates, a glossary, and useful resources.

QUESTIONS AND ANSWERS

I have put together a few questions and answers to which you can readily refer; however, it is important to review the main content of the book for more in-depth information. The following are five common questions I have received from students with answers that I hope you will find helpful.

1. Q: In order to be accepted into medical school, do you have to major in one of the sciences?

   A: No, it is not necessary to major in the sciences, although many students do so. Choose a major that interests and challenges you. Medical students should be well-rounded individuals with knowledge in various fields. You will, however, need to fulfill your science course requirements too.

2. Q: I am interested in a medical career, but I don't visualize myself working directly with patients. What options are available to me?

   A: There are many options outside of direct patient care. Doctors may choose careers with pharmaceutical or healthcare insurance companies, devote their lives to research or teaching, or become involved in public health policy. These are only a few of the possibilities. The medical field is vast, exciting, and ever-changing.

3. Q: My family will not be able to afford my medical school tuition costs. How do I begin the process of looking for financial assistance?

   A: A good place to start is by speaking to someone in your school's office of financial aid. You may be eligible for need-based aid. Other assistance may also be available in the form of talent, merit, or work aid. You may also consider applying for a scholarship or a loan. Loans will need to be repaid.

4. Q: I am a college freshman interested in applying to medical school. Do you have any advice on asking for letters of recommendation?

A: Begin the process early. Talk to your lecturers, mentors, or professors who really know you well and can speak to your knowledge, work ethic, and character. Ask if they would be willing to write letters for you. If you sense hesitation, it's best to pursue other options.

5. Q: I graduated with a degree in engineering two years ago, and I now realize this is not what I intend to do for the rest of my life. I have decided to pursue medicine instead. Will my background place me at a disadvantage?

A: Not necessarily. You will need to take the MCAT exam and fulfill the science and nonscience requirements of the medical schools to which you apply. Admissions committees are interested in well rounded, bright, motivated students from all backgrounds.

GUIDE TO THE MEDICAL SCHOOL APPLICATION PROCESS

The following is a simple ten-point plan to help you prepare for your medical school application. Details are covered in Chapters 1 through 4 as well as Chapter 6.

1. Plan your college academic curriculum.
2. Participate in extracurricular and volunteer activities—both in the medical field and outside of the medical field.
3. Research the requirements and deadlines for each medical school application.
4. Request letters of recommendation from professors/advisors/teachers who can speak to your talents, skills, and enthusiasm.
5. Apply and prepare for the Medical College Admission Test (MCAT).
6. Take the MCAT no later than the year in which you apply to medical school.
7. Send in your medical school application, including transcripts, MCAT scores, activities, letters of recommendation, and essay(s) as required.
8. Prepare for the medical school interview.
9. Keep track of deadlines.
10. Contact the office of financial aid (college and/or medical school) for information about financing your studies.

GLOSSARY

Allergist/immunologist: a physician who is a specialist in the diagnosis and treatment of allergy and disorders of the immune system

Alzheimer's disease: a form of dementia, a neurological disease that usually occurs in the elderly

Anesthesiologist: a physician who is a specialist in airway and pain management, and the care of the surgical patient

Attending: supervising physician

Autism: developmental disorder that affects social interaction and communication

Cadaver: dead body

Cardiac catheterization (heart catheterization): passage of a catheter through vessels in order to obtain information about the heart and cardiovascular system

Cardiologist: a physician who is a specialist in the treatment of disorders of the heart and cardiovascular system

CBC: complete blood count

Chernobyl: city where a nuclear power plant disaster occurred in 1986

Clavicle: collarbone

Croup: a respiratory infection usually affecting children, with symptoms including a cough that may sound like a seal's bark

ECFMG: Education Commission for Foreign Medical Graduates

Eczema (dermatitis): inflammatory skin condition

Emergency room physician: a physician who is a specialist in the care of patients with urgent or life-threatening conditions

Empyema: collection of pus in a body cavity, usually outside the lung (between the lung and chest wall)

Epiglottitis: potentially life-threatening medical condition involving inflammation of the epiglottis (structure that covers the windpipe)

Fabry disease: a genetic disorder caused by an enzyme deficiency

FLEX: United States exam for foreign medical school graduates

Gaucher disease: genetic disorder caused by deficiency of the enzyme glucocerebrosidase

Geneticist: a physician or scientist who is a specialist in the field of genetics

Genetics: the diagnosis and treatment of hereditary and genetic disorders

Grand rounds: A meeting attended by physicians and medical students in which medical problems and clinical cases are presented and discussed

Hematologist: a physician who is a specialist in the diagnosis and treatment of disorders of the blood and bone marrow

Hippocratic Oath: oath (pertaining to ethical practice) taken by new doctors upon graduation and before entering practice

Internship: first year of training after medical school (now referred to as first year residency or postgraduate level one)

JVP (jugular venous pulse or jugular venous pressure): observed pressure of the jugular vein in the neck; provides an estimate of the central venous pressure

Kawasaki disease: a disease that causes an inflammation (vasculitis) of arteries including the coronary arteries

Kwashiorkor: protein-energy malnutrition

Lyme disease: a disease caused by an infection that is transmitted by a tick bite

Marasmus: severe malnutrition usually caused by deficient intake of protein and calories

Match: National Resident Matching Program (NRMP); program that matches an applicant's residency preference with a program's preference for applicants

MCAT: Medical College Admission Test

MD: Doctor of Medicine

MD/MPH: combined degree in medicine and public health

MD/PhD: combined degree in medicine and research; equivalent to an MD and a PhD (physician-scientist)

Meningitis: inflammation of the meninges (membrane covering the brain), usually caused by infection

MRI: magnetic resonance imaging

Nebulizer: a machine that converts liquid medication into a mist so that it can be inhaled into the lungs

Neonatologist: a physician who is a specialist in the care and treatment of newborns

Obstetrician-gynecologist (ob-gyn): a physician who is a specialist in pregnancy, labor, and delivery, as well as the prevention and treatment of diseases of the female reproductive system

Oncologist: a physician who is a specialist in the diagnosis and treatment of cancers

Orthopedist: a physician who is a specialist in the treatment of injuries and disorders of the musculoskeletal system

Pathologist: a physician who is an expert in laboratory medicine as well as the analysis of body cells, tissues, fluids, and other specimens

Pediatrician: a physician who is a specialist in the treatment of infants, children, and adolescents

Petechiae: a pinpoint rash caused by bleeding from the capillary blood vessels into the skin, which may be associated with a low platelet count

Phenylketonuria (PKU): a hereditary disorder in which the body can't metabolize phenylalanine

Plastic surgeon: a surgeon who is a specialist in the treatment of disfigurement or scarring of the face or body, as well as certain skin lesions, and is qualified to perform cosmetic and reconstructive surgery

Psychiatrist: a physician who is a specialist in the treatment of mental and emotional disorders

Radiologist: a physician who is a specialist in the interpretation of radiological images for the prevention and treatment of disease and disorders

Residency: period of training (specialization) after medical school

Rickets: a disease associated with vitamin D deficiency and abnormal bone formation (ossification)

Septic bursitis: an infection of a fluid-filled sac near a joint

Stent: a device used to keep a blood vessel open

Stethoscope: a device used to auscultate (listen to) the heart and lungs

Surgeon: a physician who is a specialist in the operative (surgical) treatment of diseases, injuries, and other disorders

Tay-Sachs disease: a genetic, degenerative disorder of the nervous system caused by an enzyme deficiency

Tourniquet: a compression band or bandage

RESOURCES

Association of American Medical Colleges (AAMC)
655 K Street, NW, Ste 100
Washington, D.C. 20001-2399
(202) 828-0400
www.aamc.org

American Medical College Application Service (AMCAS)
(202) 828-0600
amcas@aamc.org
www.aamc.org/students/amcas

American Medical Student Association (AMSA)
45610 Woodland Rd, Ste 300
Sterling, VA 20166
(703) 620-6600
www.amsa.org

American Medical Women's Association (AMWA)
1100 E. Woodfield Rd, Ste 350
Schaumburg, IL 60173
(847) 517-2801
www.amwa-doc.org

Cappex
www.cappex.com
College search made simple

ECFMG
www.ecfmg.org

FastWeb Scholarship Search
www.fastweb.com

Financial Aid information page
www.finaid.org

Free Application for Federal Student Aid (FAFSA)
www.fafsa.ed.gov

MCAT Program
AAMC-MCAT
655 K Street, NW, Ste 100
Washington, D.C. 20001-2399
(202) 828-0600

National Research Mentoring Network
www.nrmnet.net

National Resident Matching Program
2121 K Street, NW, Ste 1000
Washington, D.C. 20037
(866) 653-NRMP
www.nrmp.org

National Student Loan Data System
www.nslds.ed.gov

INTERNATIONAL MEDICAL GRADUATES

International medical graduates (IMGs) have been a valuable resource and have contributed significantly to the U.S. physician workforce over the past few decades. (Akl, Elie A., et al. *The United States Physician Workforce and International Medical Graduates: Trends and Characteristics.* Society of General Internal Medicine 2007; 22: 264-268)

If you received your medical degree outside the United States or Canada, you will have to complete several important steps before being able to practice in the United States.

1. You will need to obtain ECFMG certification (see below).
2. You will have to complete an accredited residency program in the United States or Canada.
3. You must apply for a license in the state(s) in which you intend to practice.

If you are a non-U.S. resident, you must also abide by the U.S. immigration law governed by the U.S. Citizenship and Immigration Services.

ECFMG CERTIFICATION

Medical schools outside of the United States and Canada differ with respect to curriculum and educational standards. For this reason, foreign medical graduates are required to pass the Education Commission for Foreign Medical Graduates (ECFMG) certification exam to assess whether they are ready to enter programs of graduate education in the United States.

As a foreign medical graduate, you must be certified by ECFMG before you enter a U.S. residency or fellowship program that is accredited by the Accreditation Council for Graduate Medical Education (ACGME). Certification is also required before applying to take Step 3 of the United States Medical Licensing Examination (USMLE). To obtain ECFMG certification, you must meet ECFMG medical education credential requirements and pass a series of examinations.

WHO IS ELIGIBLE FOR ECFMG CERTIFICATION?

- First, you must be an international medical student or graduate.
- Your medical school must be listed in the World Directory of Medical Schools. (World Directory)
- At least four credit years at a medical school listed in the World Directory are required.
- In addition, you must supply ECFMG with copies of your medical education credentials.
- Applicants must complete both a Medical Science Examination and a Clinical Skills Examination.

This information was found on the ECFMG website on July 18, 2017.

More detailed information on ECFMG certification and the U.S. Medical Licensing Examination can be found in two booklets:

- ECFMG Information Booklet
- USMLE Bulletin of Information

You can find these books and obtain information about ECFMG requirements by visiting the following two websites:

- ECFMG website: www.ecfmg.org
- USMLE website: www.usmle.org

If you are eligible, you can begin the process of obtaining ECFMG certification by applying for an ECFMG/USMLE identification number. Thereafter, you can apply for the ECFMG examinations online at www.ecfmg.org.

APPLYING FOR GRADUATE MEDICAL EDUCATION PROGRAMS

You will find the requirements and specific information on all ACGME Programs in the Graduate Medical Education Directory. Most but not all programs require applicants to submit applications using the Electronic Residency Application Service (ERAS). ECFMG coordinates the ERAS application process of international medical graduates.

THE U.S. PHYSICIAN WORKFORCE

The percentage of international medical graduates in the United States is significant. According to the Association of American Medical Colleges: Table B3, the percentage of IMGs among 2015-2016 active residents was 24.9 percent. (Number of Active Residents, by Type of Medical School, GME Specialty, and Gender 2015-2016 Active Residents)

At one point, it was believed that there would be an overabundance of physicians in the United States, but that is no longer the case. Instead, it is projected that there will be a growing shortage of physicians. Some reasons include population growth as well as a greater number of older people requiring additional resources. Because of this shortage of U.S. physicians, we may have to rely more on foreign medical graduates and nonphysician healthcare providers, particularly in the primary care fields, which may have the highest demand. In order to address the future shortage of U.S. physicians, the Association of American Medical Colleges recommended expanding first-year medical school enrollment and increasing graduate medical education positions in 2006. To overcome the problem, it is believed that improvements in efficiency and changes in the delivery of physician services will be needed. (Dill, Michael J. and Edward S. Salsberg. Center for Workforce Studies. Association of American Medical Colleges, *The Complexities of Physician Supply and Demand: Projections Through 2025.* November, 2008.)

THE "MATCH" FOR INTERNATIONAL MEDICAL GRADUATES

International medical graduates who wish to participate with the National Resident Matching Program (NRMP), or the "Match," which matches applicants with available residency positions, must register with the NRMP.

BIBLIOGRAPHY

BOOKS

Abrams, Fredrick R. *Doctors on the Edge: Will your doctor break the rules for you?* Boulder, CO: Sentient Publications, 2006.

Ambrose, Stephen E. *Eisenhower: Soldier and President.* New York: Simon & Schuster, 1990.

Association of American Medical Colleges. The Official Guide to Medical School Admissions. How to Prepare for and Apply to Medical School. AAMC, 2017 Edition.

Carmichael, Ann G.; and Richard M. Ratzan. *Medicine: A Treasury of Art and Literature.* New York: Hugh Lauter Levin Associates, Inc., Editorial Production by Harkavy Publishing Service, Printed in China, 1991.

Chadwick, John. *The Medical Works of Hippocrates.* Translated by W.N. Mann. Oxford: Blackwell, 1950.

Donaldson Jr., Robert M., Kathleen S. Lundgren, and Howard M. Spiro. *The Yale Guide to Careers in Medicine and the Health Professions: Pathways to Medicine in the 21st Century.* New Haven and London: Yale University Press, 2003.

Freeman, Brian. *The Ultimate Guide to Choosing a Medical Specialty.* McGraw-Hill, USA: Lange Medical Books, 2004.

Groopman, Jerome. *How Doctors Think.* New York: Mariner Books, (permission granted by Houghton Mifflin Company), 2008.

Heller, Tania. *You and Your Doctor. A Guide to a Healing Relationship, with Physicians' Insights*. McFarland, 2012.

Hunter, Kathryn Montgomery. *Doctors' Stories: The Narrative Structure of Medical Knowledge*. Princeton, New Jersey: Princeton University Press, 1991.

Korda, Michael. *Ike: An American Hero*. New York: Harper Perennial, 2008.

LeClair, Mary K., Justin White, and Susan Keeter. *Three 19th-Century Women Doctors*. Syracuse, New York: Hofmann Press, 2007.

Leonard, Elizabeth D. *Yankee Women: Gender Battles in the Civil War*. New York: W.W. Norton & Company, 1994.

Miles, Steven H. *The Hippocratic Oath and the Ethics of Medicine*. New York: Oxford University Press, 2004.

Montross, Christine. *Body of Work: Meditations on Mortality from the Human Anatomy Lab*. New York: Penguin Books, 2007.

Mukherjee, Siddhartha. *The Emperor of all Maladies. A Biography of Cancer*. Scribner, 2010.

Plantz, Scott H., Nichols Y. Lorenzo, and Jesse A. Cole. *Getting into Medical School Today: The Inside Facts Every Pre-Med Should Know*. Fourth edition. Princeton, New Jersey: Peterson's, 1998.

Pories, Susan, Sachin H. Jain, and Gordon Harper. *The Soul of a Doctor*. Chapel Hill: Algonquin Books of Chapel Hill, 2006.

Porter, Roy, ed. *The Cambridge Illustrated History of Medicine*. Cambridge: Cambridge University Press, 1996.

Shem, Samuel. *The House of God*. New York: Dell Publishing, 1978. Republished 2003.

Transue, Emily R. *On Call: A Doctor's Days and Nights in Residency*. New York: St. Martin's Griffin, 2004.

ARTICLES

Akl, Elie A., et al. "The United States Physician Workforce and International Medical Graduates: Trends and Characteristics." *Society of General Internal Medicine*. Issue 2, Volume 22 (2007): 264–268.

Association of American Medical Colleges. Tuition and Student Fees for

First-Year Students. Summary Statistics for Academic Years 2012-13 through 2016-17. (February, 2017)

Association of American Medical Colleges. "(MD)^2 Monetary Decisions for Medical Doctors." www.aamc.org. 2005. Accessed January 20, 2009.

Association of American Medical Colleges. Wisenberg Brin, Dinah. Taking the Sting out of Medical School Debt. April 4, 2017. (www.aamc.org) Accessed July 9, 2017.

Association of American Medical Colleges: Table B3. Number of Active Residents, by Type of Medical School, GME Specialty, and Gender 2015-2016 Active Residents. Accessed July 18, 2017.

Committee on Pediatric Emergency Medicine. "Pediatric Care Recommend-ations for Freestanding Urgent Care Facilities." *American Academy of Pediatrics: Pediatrics*. Issue 1, Volume 116 (July 2005): 258–60.

Dill, Michael J., and Edward S. Salsberg. "The Complexities of Physician Supply and Demand: Projections through 2025." *Association of American Medical Colleges: Center for Workforce Studies* (November 2008).

Jones, M., Leslie Douglas Jr., K. Laurel, and Gail A. McGuinness, eds. "Residency Review and Redesign in *Pediatrics*: New (and Old) Questions." Pediatrics. Supplement 1, Volume 123 (January 2009).

United States Census Bureau. Detailed Languages Spoken at Home and Ability to Speak English for the Population 5 Years and Over: 2009-2013. (Release Date: October 2015) www.census.gov Accessed July 14, 2017.

Whelan, Gerald P., et al. "The Changing Pool of International Medical Graduates Seeking Certification Training in U.S. Graduate Medical Education Programs." *American Medical Association* (Reprinted) JAMA, Issue 9, Volume 288 (September 2002): 1079–1084.

INDEX

A

AAMC. *See* Association of American Medical Colleges (AAMC)

AAMC Curriculum Directory, 30

ABMS. *See* American Board of Medical Specialties (ABMS)

Accreditation Council for Graduate Medical Education (ACGME), 77, 203

ACGME. *See* Accreditation Council for Graduate Medical Education (ACGME)

advisor(s), premedical, for helping students with medical school admission requirements and medical school applications, 71

Albany Hospital, Albany, New York, 163

Albert Einstein, Philadelphia, Pennsylvania, 162

Albert Lasker Award for Clinical Medical Research, 186

allergist/immunologist, defined, 196

allergy(ies), described, 154

allergy/immunology, 153–55

    advances in, 155

    described, 153

    routine and lifestyle in, 154–55

    training for, 153

Allison, Brian, 50–52

Alzheimer's disease, 118

    defined, 196

AMCAS. *See* American Medical College Application Service (AMCAS)

American Academy of Child and Adolescent Psychiatry, 164

American Academy of Pediatrics, 157

American Board of Medical Specialties (ABMS), 78

American College of Medical Genetics, 104

American College of Surgeons, 160

American Medical Association, 157

    FREIDA of, 78

American Medical College Application Service (AMCAS), 26, 34–37

American Medical Student Association (AMSA), 30

American Osteopathic Association, 28

AMSA. *See* American Medical Student Association (AMSA)

anencephaly, 132

anesthesiologist

    defined, 196

    described, 143

anesthesiology, 143–45

    advances in, 145

    advice for students, 145

    challenges facing, 143–45

    clinical situation, 143–44

    described, 143

    settings for, 145

    training for, 143

angiography, coronary, CT, 139

angioplasty, balloon, 121

Army Human Resources Command, Medical Corp Branch at, 151

art of medicine, 82

associate dean, interview with, 35–37

Association of American Medical Colleges (AAMC), 25, 30, 204

    on EDP, 34

    on medical school first year tuition, 66

attending, defined, 196

autism, defined, 196

B

balloon angioplasty, 121

Barnard, Christiaan, 4

ABOUT THE AUTHOR

Tania Heller, MD, is a board-certified pediatrician, the former medical director of the Washington Center for Eating Disorders and Adolescent Obesity in Maryland, and an Independent Medical School Admissions Consultant (see www.taniahellerconsulting.com). She is the author of four other books: *You and Your Doctor: A Guide to a Healing Relationship, with Physicians' Insights*; *Overweight: A Handbook for Teens and Parents*; *Eating Disorders: A Handbook for Teens, Families and Teachers*; and *Pregnant! What Can I Do?: A Guide for Teenagers*, published by McFarland.